The Power of Patient Stories

Learning Moments In Medicine

By

Paul F. Griner, MD

ISBN: 1478178302

ISBN 13: 9781478178309

Library of Congress Control Number: 2012912028
CreateSpace, North Charleston, SC

Dedication

To my late wife, Mimi, and to Laura, Paul, and Margaret

Table of Contents

PART ONE

About Ethics and Professionalism in Medicine

PART TWO

The Importance of Good Bedside Skills:
Listening, Observing, Examining

PART THREE

Learning Moments from Other Stories

PART FOUR

Key Challenges for Today's Medical Schools

Foreward

Education of physicians begins in medical school and continues throughout one's professional life. When educating medical students, the importance of strong interpersonal relationships must be emphasized. However, advances in medical technology have made relating to patients more difficult. This is not a new problem.

"When one considers the amazing progress of science in its relation to medicine during the last thirty years, and the enormous mass of scientific material which must be made available to the modern physician, it is not surprising that the schools have tended to concern themselves more and more with this phase of the educational problem."[i] So wrote Francis Peabody in 1927 regarding students at Harvard Medical School.

Medical practice has become more impersonal. There is less time to see patients, more interaction with computers in the presence of patients, and an increasing dependence on subspecialists. Ethical issues arise with the expansion of complex diagnostic and therapeutic procedures. To meet these problems, medical schools have expanded teaching to help students improve interpersonal skills and solve ethical problems.

Despite contemporary challenges, medicine has maintained its basic character. Patients seek help in treating their illnesses, and physicians provide that help. Knowledge, judgment, and sound clinical reasoning are all necessary. A positive relationship with the patient is key to the successful resolution of problems. The medical interview, along with genuine concern for the patient, helps establish this relationship. Medical educators benefit students by observing their interviews and physical diagnostic skills. The fact that physician teachers have less time with students should not deter them from observing student interactions with patients. The teacher should always strive to be a positive role model.

Stories have universal appeal because they dominate our culture in personal reminiscences, literature, movies, and the media. Medical case histories are very effective teaching tools. In *The Power of Patient Stories*, Paul Griner tells of his many experiences with patient care. Throughout these case studies, one witnesses his positive patient relationships and how he strives to do what is best for each person. When a physician does not give a patient time to describe symptoms, substitutes advanced technology for clinical skills, and jumps to conclusions, the patient suffers.

The case reports in this book illustrate many problems. Included are patients whose confidentiality is compromised and whose privacy is invaded. Sometimes decisions have to be made in the patient's best interest even when others disagree. There are special circumstances where judgment may alter conventional therapy. Should one report a physician who is incompetent? Is it right to accelerate death when there is terminal suffering? The finding of missed diagnoses is described. Cases illustrate the value of physical diagnosis and the importance of following patients in order to understand their illnesses. Knowing what to do with bad behavior is another issue. At the end of each case report, questions are asked about the decisions that have been made, especially where treatment is controversial.

One can learn from these stories how to communicate with and treat patients. The fundamental principle underlying patient care was stated eighty-five years ago by Francis Peabody: "One of the essential qualities of the clinician is interest in humanity, for the secret of the care of the patient is in caring for the patient."[ii]

William L. Morgan, MD

Preface

Between wisdom and medicine there is no gulf fixed; in fact, medicine possesses all the qualities that make for wisdom.

HIPPOCRATES

This book is meant to be both educational and entertaining. It is written primarily for students of the health professions—medical, nursing, pharmacy—and health administration students. It consists of patients' stories I collected throughout my career in medicine. Most of the stories provided a learning moment for me. Hopefully the same will be true for those who read this book. The remaining stories are interesting, often poignant, vignettes of the kind that physicians have stored in their memory banks, the result of many years of patient care. As such, the book may be of interest to a general audience as well.

More than fifty stories are presented, reflecting my experiences over a fifty-eight-year career in medicine. Medical school included an extra—and extraordinary—year as a student fellow in pathology. Residency training was followed by a tour of duty in the air force as a hematologist. Most of my subsequent career was spent at the University of Rochester School of Medicine, first as an internist and hematologist, then as president of Strong Memorial Hospital. I completed my career at the Massachusetts General Hospital, where I had been a resident fifty years earlier. Few physicians have had the opportunity to share stories from so many different perspectives.

Most of the vignettes in this book occurred during the 1950s and 1960s, prior to what we now refer to as modern medicine. Patients then were often hospitalized to determine the cause of elusive symptoms, such as persistent unexplained fever or weight loss. Today, patients are hospitalized principally for treatment of a problem already well established. Fifty years ago, imaging was limited to conventional x-rays. Laboratory tests were not particularly sophisticated; automated tests such as the SMA-6 and SMA-12 were just arriving on the scene. Computed tomography (CT), magnetic resonance imaging (MRI), and nuclear and positron emission tomography (PET) scans had not yet been developed.

Autopsies were performed on most patients who died in the hospital to determine the cause of death or to confirm suspected diagnoses. Endoscopes to examine the bronchial system, esophagus, stomach, and colon were rigid steel tubes, uncomfortable for patients and thus not used as frequently as today's flexible fiber-optic scopes. Antibiotics were limited in number. None were particularly effective against penicillin-resistant staphylococci. Poliomyelitis had just been eradicated. Tuberculosis was still a common disease. Medical specialties such as hematology, oncology, endocrinology, and gastroenterology were just being developed.

In this era of medicine, a premium was placed upon the physician's ability to capture as much information as possible from a comprehensive patient history and a thorough physical examination. Indeed, studies have shown that among patients coming to their physician with an undiagnosed problem, as many as 80–90 percent of diagnoses could be suspected or confirmed by a careful history, and another 10 percent from the physical examination.[iii] Tests were used principally to confirm, not to find, a diagnosis.

With the remarkable technology now available to facilitate the diagnosis and treatment of patients, medical educators have devoted less time to the fine points of "bedside medicine"—the taking of a thorough history and performance of a good physical exam. The result is that many medical students are seriously deficient in these skills.[iv]

There are many reasons why physicians need to develop and refine these skills. First, it goes without saying that the confidence of the patient in his or her physician is of crucial importance. The patient views the performance of a thorough history and physical examination as an indication of a careful physician.

Second, the ready availability of sophisticated tests and procedures leads to their overuse. In an era of escalating and unaffordable health care costs, it is imperative that physicians be more discriminating in the use of these tools. Of even greater importance is the harm to patients that may result from the overuse of tests. All tests have some risk of falsely identifying a problem (false positive tests). Many studies have shown that the excessive availability and overuse of diagnostic technology can be harmful to patients.[v]

Third, the practice of medicine has become global. Many physicians (and students) elect to spend time in underdeveloped countries, providing valuable services to patients in settings where sophisticated tests and procedures are not available. Sound medical history and physical examination skills are essential for the proper care of these patients. Medical students who return from such experiences have learned, for the first time, the importance of these skills.

Finally, the experience of making a diagnosis with only one's eyes and ears is the essence of the art of medicine.

Forty or fifty years ago, with far fewer tests and procedures, the pace of hospital medicine was much slower. The slower pace permitted the physician to spend more time with patients, to understand them as people, and to learn their hopes and dreams. When I was an intern, I got into the habit of making rounds twice a day. Morning rounds were all business—evaluating the progress of patients, setting goals for the day, and writing the appropriate orders. Evening rounds were "social" rounds. They were an opportunity to get to know the patients, to learn about their families, their dreams, their fears. It provided an extraordinary opportunity for intimacy and honesty. I treasured evening rounds, as did the patients. My medical students were impressed with this approach to medical care. Some copied it in their later years.

This was also my habit during my years as a hematologist. If anything, evening rounds with these patients were to them the most important of the day. Most patients had malignant diseases that would kill them. Acute leukemia and Hodgkin's disease headed the list. How courageous these patients were—and how open when given the opportunity. We talked about family, sports, politics. The topic was not important. What *was* important was the chance for them to disengage from the concerns of their awful diseases for a few minutes. It was a chance for human interaction on an intensely personal level. As much as I learned about them, they learned about me, my work, and my family. Evening rounds were priceless. Sadly, these moments have been lost in the complexity and pace of work in today's world of medicine.

Medicine today is a growth industry. Health care consumes about 18 percent of our GNP, so there is a great deal of money to be made by those who produce medical products, insure people's health, and provide health services. In this environment, physicians may lose sight of the importance of being a professional. The late Supreme Court justice Louis Brandeis eloquently defined the word *profession* as "an occupation for which the necessary preliminary training is intellectual in character, involving knowledge and to some extent learning, as distinguished from mere skill; second, it is an occupation which is pursued largely for others, and not merely for one's self; third, it is an occupation in which the amount of financial return is not the accepted measure of success."[vi]

Professionalism and sound clinical skills mark the good physician. It is with this in mind that I present these stories and the lessons learned from them.

Acknowledgments

I benefited from the comments and suggestions of a number of people who reviewed various iterations of this book. As medical students, Christopher Chang, Michael Hunter, Ted Ryser, and Michael Feldman read the stories and provided comment. Their perspectives and feedback were invaluable. My daughter, Dr. Laura Hill, gave me good advice about context. My son, Paul Griner Jr., an accomplished author, was a great help in every phase of the book's development. Laura Strauss gave an editorial review that helped the book achieve readiness for publication as did the editorial staff at Createspace.com. Finally, my wife, Margaret, saw the book through the eyes of the general reader and her practical suggestions were always helpful.

Introduction

This book deals with matters of ethics, professionalism, and the importance of sound clinical skills. Abstract knowledge gained from texts and papers on these subjects is made real through the telling of patients' stories. Most of these stories resulted in a significant learning moment for me. Many caused me to pause and reflect on the values that define ethical and professional behavior and to ask myself whether I was adhering to these values. Others reinforced the importance of the skills of history-taking and physical examination and an understanding of the whole patient, the hallmarks of the education I received at the University of Rochester School of Medicine. These stories are just as relevant today as they were fifty years ago. Indeed, many would say more so.

The stories in Part One of the book point out how often issues of ethics and professionalism occur in the practice of medicine. Truthfulness, justice, dignity, and confidentiality are among the values that define ethical behavior, and the stories give the student an appreciation of how the physician is challenged to acknowledge and uphold these values in the day-to-day care of patients. Similarly, the stories about professionalism invite the student to reflect on them, share feelings about them, and thus help anchor the values that characterize the good physician.

Part Two consists of stories that emphasize the importance of good bedside skills: the art of listening, observation, and examination. These skills are poorly developed among many of today's medical students. Too often, technology trumps valuable information that can be gleaned from the hospital bedside or the clinic examination room. It is distressing to hear a resident physician order a "blue-plate special" of laboratory tests on an acutely ill patient before ever seeing him or her. The stories in this part of the book point to the importance of listening, observing, and examining in achieving early diagnosis, using laboratory tests mostly to confirm, not to seek, diagnoses.

The stories in Part Three help the student understand the remarkable nature of humans: how their bodies work naturally to heal themselves of illness, how courage and humor in the face of fatal illnesses help the patient cope, and how faith and attitude make such a difference in patient outcomes.

The medicine of today is fast-paced and technologically driven. Too often, it is organized around physicians and facilities, not patients. The last part of the book suggests strategies that should help students maintain balance in their care of patients, balance that will allow them to apply the marvels of modern medicine, accommodate pressures for cost control, and not lose track of the humanistic aspects of patient care.

PART ONE

About Ethics and Professionalism in Medicine

Values that commonly apply to medical ethics include truthfulness and honesty, justice (distribution of health resources and the decision of who gets what treatment), dignity, confidentiality, and "first, do no harm" (primum non nocere).

Epstein and Hundert described professional competence as "the habitual and judicious use of communication, knowledge, technical skills, clinical reasoning, emotions, values, and reflection in daily practice for the benefit of the individual and community being served."[vii]

The stories in this section of the book (chapters 1 through 21) reinforce the need to be constantly mindful of the challenges to ethical and professional behavior that occur in the day-to-day practice of medicine.

CHAPTER 1

The Protective Parent

Truth is the daughter of time, not of authority.

FRANCIS BACON

One Friday evening in the fall of 1967, I was called to the emergency room of a rural hospital to see the patient of a local physician who was out of town at a meeting. The patient was a twenty-one-year-old married woman, a senior at a local college. She was experiencing considerable abdominal pain. She had had acute lymphoblastic leukemia as a child. Treatment had resulted in a complete remission. Recently, she had relapsed and was again under treatment. A common side effect of one of her chemotherapy medications was abdominal discomfort.

The patient's mother intercepted me before I saw the patient to let me know that her daughter did not know of the diagnosis of leukemia and I was not to tell her. I asked her to explain the situation further. She indicated that when the diagnosis of acute leukemia was initially made, she kept this diagnosis from her daughter. She requested that everyone involved with her care agree to tell the daughter that her problem was an unusual anemia. Apparently, they complied. When the leukemia went into remission, the mother considered this chapter of her daughter's life closed.

When the daughter fell in love, became engaged, and began to make plans for a wedding, the mother did not share the previous diagnosis with either her daughter or the fiancé. When I asked the mother why she hadn't made the disclosure, she responded, "I had enough problems to deal with. I didn't need any more." The mother then asked where I lived. When I replied, she said, "Oh, dear! A number of my daughter's friends live in that area. I'm concerned that they will hear of her diagnosis from you." I was astounded and insulted. The mother's preoccupation with the need to protect her daughter from the diagnosis of her leukemia was so great that she was unable to recognize that I would be committed to hold all information about patients as confidential.

Questions:*

1. *What would you have said to the mother when she told you not to tell her daughter?*
2. *What would you have done in this situation? Would you have told the patient about her leukemia? Why or why not?*
3. *Can you think of at least two reasons why the mother may not want to share the news of the diagnosis with her daughter?*
4. *At what age does the patient have the right to know her diagnosis?*
5. *Have you ever witnessed a similar situation? What was the final result?*

*(Note that the author's responses to the questions posed at the end of each story are recorded in the back section of the book under "R*esponses to Questions*")

People who hear this story are shocked at how presumptuous it was for the patient's mother to withhold the diagnosis of leukemia from her daughter. Her insistence that the daughter not be told of her disease began a pattern of living with an ever-bigger lie for almost seven years. How was it that the father supported this charade? Once one commits to the initial lie, the need to sustain it may reach an extreme; witness the mother's frantic preoccupation with keeping this secret over a period of years.

It is important to note that in the middle of the last century, it was common to withhold bad news from patients for fear they would decompensate emotionally, even physically. In the 1960s, only 10 percent of physicians believed it was correct to tell a patient of a fatal diagnosis. [viii] Today, of course, we know that to be not so. Surveys have shown that 90 percent of patients wish to know what the future holds for them, and almost all physicians feel that they should be told. Patients trust their physicians to be empathetic and supportive, yet direct and honest. Indeed, there have been patients who, after receiving news of an incurable cancer, have thanked their doctor, showing more concern for the doctor than themselves, saying, "It must have been hard for you to tell me this."

Some medical ethicists argue that a physician may withhold information from a patient if, in his or her opinion, the information would be damaging to the patient, someone who, for example, is seriously depressed. This action by the physician is referred to as "therapeutic privilege." Courts have ruled, however, that if a patient is capable of consenting to treatment, he or she must receive the appropriate information.[ix]

Forty years ago, when this patient was being treated, many patients with acute lymphoblastic leukemia entered a remission but few were cured. Today, the cure rate is almost 90 percent. Indeed, the leukemic cells may be so sensitive to treatment that caution is called for when initiating therapy. A white blood cell count of 100,000/uL may fall to less than 5,000 overnight after a single treatment, placing the patient at risk for complications of massive cell death, such as very high potassium and uric acid levels. Wouldn't it be wonderful if all such cancers were so responsive?

CHAPTER 2

On Being Transparent

Medicine sometimes snatches away health, sometimes gives it.

Ovid

One of the first things I learned after being appointed president of Strong Memorial Hospital was to deal openly with patients and families (and the community) when mistakes were made. A fatal error was made on a six-year-old patient with a defect in bowel function who was hospitalized for severe constipation. He was given a dose of neostigmine (a drug that stimulates peristaltic activity) that was ten times the normal dose—a decimal point error made by the resident who ordered the drug. Instead of 0.4 mg the patient received 4 mg. Tragically, he died the same day from the overdose.

My director of human resources advised me to hold a press conference, immediately, to announce our mistake. I did so. The conference lasted for two hours. Reporters asked why the resident and nurse had not been fired.

I explained that both were highly regarded and that the problem was a "system" problem, not a problem of an incompetent physician or nurse. We should have had in place a fail-safe arrangement to prevent such a mistake. Today, hospitals have electronic medication-error-avoidance systems. We had no such system in 1984. I indicated to the reporters that we would be examining the medication administration procedures in place from the point the medicine was ordered to the time it was given and would put in place a procedure or procedures to ensure that such an error could not be possible again.

The reporters were impressed with our prompt acknowledgment that we had made a tragic mistake, costing the life of a young boy, even before his death was recorded in the papers and on television. The press coverage was balanced and fair. The hospital's reputation was maintained, indeed even enhanced, as the result of our actions.

When we tracked the process in place from the ordering to administration of a drug, we found there was an average of 104 steps! This was astounding. The steps included those on the patient floor (physician order, secretary transcribing the order), communication to the pharmacy, dozens of steps in the pharmacy, transportation of the medicine to the floor, receipt and recording of the receipt, and finally administration to the patient. Despite, or perhaps because of, all these steps, the error had not been prevented. The KISS principle (keep it simple, stupid) was clearly called for. We reduced the number of steps to fifty-four.

Today, most hospitals have automated drug-ordering systems that would identify the error in the drug dose typed in by the physician, interrupt the ordering sequence, and bring the error to the attention of the physician.

This episode contrasted sharply with an experience I had with a wealthy patient from Geneva, Switzerland, who traveled to the States each year for a comprehensive examination. Before coming to Rochester from his overseas flight, his habit was to spend a few days in New York City visiting friends. On one such annual trip, he was hit by a bicyclist, fell, and fractured his pelvis. He was admitted to a well-known hospital in the city and spent three weeks convalescing, in bed the entire time. I received a call from him at that point asking to be transferred to Strong Memorial Hospital in Rochester. He was unhappy with his care, indicating that no one seemed to be attending to him. We arranged the transfer. I saw him the afternoon of his transfer and was astounded to find that he had a pressure ulcer on his heel an inch deep! How could this have happened? The ulcer would not heal. He had peripheral arterial insufficiency. It was necessary for me to secure a vascular surgeon to perform arterial bypass surgery. The surgery was successful. Good blood flow was established and, over a period of weeks, the ulcer healed completely.

I was furious with the poor care he had received at the hospital in New York City. I wrote a letter to the president of the facility. Some weeks later, after not receiving a response, I called his office. I was transferred to the hospital lawyer. I indicated the reason for the call and asked why I had not received a response. He said, "Oh, we would never acknowledge a mistake, we might get sued." I replied icily that we did things differently in upstate New York. We acknowledged mistakes promptly so we *wouldn't* be sued.

It is important that mistakes be disclosed to patients for a number of reasons. First, hospitals that practice full disclosure may experience a reduction in their malpractice costs.[10] Second, the reputation of the hospital and its medical staff may be enhanced. Finally, and most importantly, the mistake provides an opportunity to determine the reason and to implement steps to ensure that it does not happen again. It is essential that physicians in training as well as students in other health professions understand the importance of this point.

It is remarkable to note how many patients walk out of hospitals today with a new lease on life resulting from the growth of medical knowledge and technology—patients with repaired joints, improved circulation to their hearts and brains to reduce the risk of heart attack and stroke, cancers cured, and the like. Yet these miracles of modern medicine don't occur without risk. In 1964, an article appeared in the Annals of Internal Medicine with the title "The Hazards of Hospitalization" detailing the frequency and types of unexpected patient events that occurred on the medical floors of the Yale-New Haven Hospital in New Haven, Connecticut.[xi] The chief resident in medicine had had his interns report on each and every event that resulted in harm to patients for a full year. The findings included medication errors, other treatment complications, falls, drug interactions, transfusion problems, and complications of diagnostic tests among types of adverse events. Today, these problems are still with us. In a highly regarded report by the Institute of Medicine of the National Academy of Sciences, published in 2002, it was estimated that as many as 98,000 preventable deaths occurred each year in US hospitals.[xii] Aggressive approaches to the improvement of quality are reducing this number, but the advice of many is that if a family member is hospitalized, it would be well for someone from the family to always be present.

Questions:

1. *List some of the adverse events you have observed among hospitalized patients. Which were preventable?*
2. *What criteria would you use to decide whether an error is serious enough to inform the patient that a mistake was made?*

CHAPTER 3

Not Enough Respirators

A physician is obligated to consider more than a diseased organ, more even than the whole man—he must view the man in his world.

HARVEY CUSHING

Halfway through my internship year, I was on one of the male medical wards of the Massachusetts General Hospital when the influenza epidemic of 1960 hit Boston. Soon we were inundated with patients with pneumonia. Most were men with chronic lung disease from smoking, their lungs susceptible to complications of the flu. Our normal patient census was about eighteen; during the two months of the flu epidemic, we averaged forty patients. Since the ward had only twenty beds, half our patients were scattered throughout other areas of the hospital—including the gynecology service! Our patients were very sick. At least half required portable respirators to assist their breathing. We had only eight or ten respirators, however. It was up to us to choose which patients would receive a respirator and which would not. My resident and I developed a decision-making process we could both agree on. In addition to severity of illness, other factors we considered were age, predicted quality of life after recovery, family structure, and likelihood of survival of the acute episode with the addition of a respirator. We allocated respirators according to this homemade set of determinants.

One morning on rounds, I observed one of my patients drinking his urine. He was one of the recipients of a respirator, to no avail. He was delirious, his blood oxygen level was low, and his carbon dioxide level very high—the highest I had ever witnessed. He died later that day; so much for our decision algorithm. We fell back to the assignment of respirators on the basis of a "gut feel" about the patient and his environment.

During the two months of the influenza outbreak, 50 percent of our patients died. We went through this terrible period like automatons. There was little privacy to be had on the ward A green pull curtain was all that separated one patient from another. We had a two-bed "annex" adjacent to the ward where we transferred patients who were terminally ill so that they might die in peace with their families present. Once it became known by the ward patients that a move to the annex was an indication of imminent death, no patient would accept a transfer to the room.

It was the tradition (and responsibility) for interns and residents to present every death that occurred during their time on duty at "Allen Street rounds." The chief of medicine, other senior physicians, and all interns and residents attended these rounds where the quality of the care we provided was reviewed and critiqued. Most interns would present at Allen Street rounds once or twice a year. I presented at Allen Street rounds *every week* for the next year!

During World War I, injured soldiers were met at the battlefield hospital by a medical officer who assigned them levels of urgency according to his estimate of the chances of survival. Those whose survival might depend on immediate treatment received the highest priority. Next were those who were expected to survive. Those not expected to survive received just supportive care, usually morphine to relieve pain and fear. Medical triage was thus established. My partner's and my attempt at a more explicit formula for assigning patients to respirators failed as an alternate to intuitive decision-making. In retrospect, we probably were subconsciously using the formula to assuage our guilt over making decisions about who might live and who would likely not, a heady responsibility for young physicians. It would have been helpful if I had followed and recorded the outcomes of patients who did and did not receive respirators and my feelings about them.

Questions:

1. *Faced with fewer respirators than were needed, how would you arrive at decisions about who would receive a respirator and who would not?*
2. *Can these kinds of decisions be made without involving the patient or his or her family?*
3. *Today, one can predict the survival of critically ill patients using various physiologic and biochemical measurements. In your opinion, what chance of survival would merit the use of a ventilator to sustain a patient—50 percent, 10 percent, 1 percent?*

CHAPTER 4

Just One More Week

To array a man's will against his sickness is the supreme art of medicine.

HENRY WARD BEECHER

One Saturday afternoon, I received a call from a local couple. Would I be willing to see their son, a sophomore in college? It seemed that while dragging furniture up a stairway to his college dorm, he collapsed. The college infirmary noted that he was very pale, drew a blood sample, and found that he was severely anemic and, in addition, deficient in both white cells and platelets. Arrangements were made to have him fly to Rochester, and we admitted him to the hospital that same afternoon. Soon after admission, we obtained a sample of bone marrow. It was literally empty of blood-forming cells; no precursors of red cells, white cells, or platelets. This condition is known as aplastic anemia.

Most often, the cause of aplastic anemia is unknown. In some cases, an adverse effect of a prescribed drug is the cause. In 1970, when this patient was hospitalized, the antibiotic chloramphenicol was known be associated with aplastic anemia. At the time, chloramphenicol was administered to patients who had staph infections that were resistant to penicillin. When semisynthetic penicillin derivatives were developed, the need for chloramphenicol evaporated. Eventually it was removed from the market as a drug that posed an unnecessary risk. As it turns out, the patient had spent the summer touring Mexico. On one occasion, he'd developed an intense bout of diarrhea and gone to a local physician. The physician prescribed chloramphenicol. We presumed that the drug was responsible for the patient's aplastic anemia.

For about a month, we observed the patient in the hospital to determine whether the disease might be transient. During that time, we treated him with frequent transfusions of red cells, white cells, and platelets. The local blood bank had to work very hard to identify enough people willing to donate their platelets or white cells. Such donors would have to go to a blood bank and sit for four to five hours while blood flowed out of one arm and back in the other. Blood flowing out would be rich in red cells, platelets, and white cells. Blood flowing in would have either the platelets or white cells missing, having been "spun off" by a differential centrifuge in the process. During this month in the hospital, the patient had repeated infections requiring intravenous antibiotics.

After it became clear that the patient was not going to have a spontaneous reversal of the aplastic anemia, we were stuck. We would not be able to identify enough donors to transfuse him endlessly. We became aware of a case of a child with aplastic anemia at Johns Hopkins Hospital who had recovered after receiving cyclophosphamide, a chemotherapeutic drug used most often in patients with Hodgkin's disease and non-Hodgkin's lymphomas. The treatment was purely experimental, based on a hypothesis that the aplastic anemia was an autoimmune reaction and that a drug known to be useful in such disorders might be effective. We discussed this option among ourselves and then with the patient and his parents.

It was clear that he would die within a few months at most, either from an infection or from bleeding. We would not be able to keep up with daily demands for these cells indefinitely. It was equally likely that he would die from the large dose of cyclophosphamide that would have to be given if his bone marrow did not recover spontaneously. The patient and family were of one mind. They wanted to pursue the chance for marrow recovery through the experimental approach with cyclophosphamide. We agreed that we would do everything possible to keep him alive for the next six weeks. If he did not respond by then, we would stop supporting him with replacement blood cells and leave the rest to nature.

The patient was given a huge dose of cyclophosphamide, larger by far than any I had ever given anyone else. He continued to deteriorate, losing some forty pounds and with evidence of multiple skin abscesses and urinary tract infections. Each day, we administered platelets and white blood cells. Red cell transfusions were needed about once every ten days. He was uncomfortable and depressed, usually curled up in bed in a fetal position. About a week before Christmas, his mother came to me and asked us to stop keeping him alive, that he had given up and she could not stand to see him suffer further. We walked into the patient's room together and I asked whether they would consent to one more week of white cell and platelet transfusions. One more week would bring us to the six-week point, the time we had originally agreed to. Both the mother and the patient agreed to an additional week.

A few days later, on Christmas morning, the blood count showed a few of the patient's own white blood cells. Within days, his white cell and platelet counts were rising. I vividly recall seeing him on New Year's evening, lying in bed with his many skin abscesses healing, having a beer with some of his buddies, knowing that he was on the mend. What a fabulous feeling for all of us. Two weeks later, he was able to leave the hospital. He was generating enough of all the blood cell lines to be on his own.

Within another month, all his blood counts were normal, his infections had all cleared, he had gained back twenty-five pounds, and he was talking about returning to school. He completed college, eventually returning to Rochester where he married and settled down. He became a strong proponent of the Rochester Regional Blood Bank. During his illness, one donor in particular had come to the blood bank three times a week to donate white cells to my patient. The patient eventually hooked up with this donor, and they became very close.

This was the first published case of successful treatment of aplastic anemia with an immunosuppressive drug.[xiii] The story reflects the dilemma we face daily in this country—whether to spend an enormous amount of resources on one patient in the remote likelihood that he or she will benefit or to use that money for preventive and other services for a large number of people. This patient's hospital bill was about a quarter of a million dollars. In 1970 dollars, that was a huge amount of money. It would have been a substantial nest egg for the local Department of Health to use to benefit the local population.

While the physician's first responsibility is to his or her patient, each of us needs to consider these economic tradeoffs as we grapple with decisions about whether to keep alive a patient who has little chance of surviving, let alone returning to a functional life. Cases that pose ethical dilemmas arise every day; rarely is there a "right way." Age is certainly a consideration. Few would argue with the premise that, all things considered, limited resources favor their use among younger patients.

The dilemmas can cause confusion and anxiety among young physicians. To address this issue, family medicine residents at Columbia/Presbyterian Hospital in New York City receive a narrative ethics curriculum. They write about patients whose cases involve ethical considerations and then share them with their colleagues. Residents find this approach rewarding and useful, helping them in their future actions with ethically challenging patient problems.

Questions:

1. *What is an advance directive? In the absence of such a directive, is a physician or nurse obligated to do everything possible to sustain life?*
2. *What are the steps needed to obtain informed consent to use an experimental drug?*

CHAPTER 5

Invasion of Privacy

The best way to find out if you can trust somebody is to trust them.

ERNEST HEMINGWAY

One day the parents of a fourteen-year-old girl brought her to my office and asked if I would perform a pelvic examination to determine whether she was a virgin. They had intercepted and read a letter from a boyfriend who was in the army at the time. From the letter, the parents inferred that their daughter had had intercourse with the boyfriend.

The parents' appearance and demeanor reminded me of the painting *American Gothic* by Grant Wood, of the Kansas farmer and his wife standing in front of their home, he holding a pitchfork.

After recovering from the shock of the parents' invasion of the privacy of this young woman, I accompanied her to an exam room, closed the door, and asked her to sit on the examining table. I took her pulse. It was about 120/minute, her hands were cold, and she was shaking slightly. She was terrified that I would examine her and find that she was not virginal. I relieved her fear by informing her that I would not be doing an examination and that I would tell her parents that she was indeed still a virgin. I added that the suspicion shown by her mother and father pointed to the need for more effective communication among them. I gave her a few pointers about breaking the ice to improve communication and what she might do to gain their trust.

We returned to my office where the parents were waiting. I told them that their daughter was likely still a virgin. I expressed my concern over what I regarded as an invasion of her privacy. It was all I could do not to show my disgust over their behavior.

Questions:

1. *Can you tell whether a fourteen-year-old girl is virginal?*
2. *What would you have said to the parents of this patient?*

Some would say that parents have the right to read their children's mail if they feel that the child is at risk of being harmed by the person with whom they are corresponding or is going against personal or religious principles. The rationale for the former is clearer to most than the latter. To the contrary, some clergy have taken the position that if parents feel that their child's behavior is not in line with the teachings of their faith and may be influenced by whoever is writing to him or her, the parents may read the child's mail to determine whether the behavior is compliant.

When the issue is confidentiality of medical information, the legal status of minors is a complex one. Parental consent is not required for minors to obtain contraceptives. There are a number of legal precedents that permit contraceptives to be prescribed without parental consent. One of the most interesting occurred in the state of Connecticut. Prior to 1965, Connecticut had a statute that made it a criminal offense to prescribe or use contraceptives. A member of Planned Parenthood of Connecticut and a physician who prescribed contraceptives were arrested and fined for giving unmarried couples advice on contraception. A lawsuit was subsequently brought by Planned Parenthood and the physician challenging the constitutionality of the Connecticut statute. It was indeed found to be unconstitutional, as was the finding for a similar law in the state of Massachusetts that was appealed all the way to the United States Supreme Court. The court found for the plaintiffs, noting that "minors had a fundamental right to choose... whether to bear or beget a child."[xiv]

In most states, however, parental notification *is* required when a minor is seeking an abortion. Some minors discuss the intent to have an abortion with their parents. Many who do not are often abused children who fear physical violence if they tell the parents of their pregnancy. Still others don't want their parents to know that they have disregarded the expectations of their families.

Contraceptive services and abortion remain very much on the front burner of debate in this country. Health policy decisions continue to be lightning rods for this debate as indicated by the divergent views of conservatives and liberals over the 2012 federal requirement that employers pay for contraceptive services for their employees.

CHAPTER 6

Exposed

No man is a good doctor who has never been sick himself.

CHINESE PROVERB

Sometime in 1994, while I was still president of the hospital, I showed up in my business suit for a visit with a dermatologist. She had me undress for a full skin exam. No shorts or undershirt. I was given a gown to put on. It looked like the gown I had used forty years earlier when I was in the emergency room with a kidney stone my freshman year in medical school. The gown was torn where the buttons met over the right shoulder and it kept slipping off. Throughout the examination, I felt vulnerable and humiliated.

The next day, just before our weekly meeting, I had my management team assemble in the conference room next to my office. Alone in my office, I took off all my clothes and donned the gown, then entered the conference room. I was met with a gasp of surprise. I sat down and said, "Let me tell you a little story." I then proceeded to describe my dermatology visit the day before and the humiliation I felt. I pointed out how vulnerable patients feel in a hospital setting, how much they are at the mercy of the "system." I reminded them of the motto, to heal when possible, to relieve often, and to comfort always. We discussed the importance of respecting patients' values, their autonomy, and their privacy; of keeping them informed of their clinical status and prognosis; of involving them in medical decisions; and of communicating with their families as well. Most importantly, we talked about the need to do everything possible to help patients maintain their dignity under trying circumstances

This brief interlude made a great impression on the management team. We decided to do something about patient gowns. One of the members of the management team was assigned the task of finding out more about our hospital gowns. A few weeks later, he reported back, indicating that the hospital had twelve different types of gowns and that none met our expectations of comfort, ease of use, or decorum. We reduced the number of gowns by 75 percent and changed vendors in order to meet our new criteria.

It is now fifteen years after that event and the members of the management team, wherever they are, still talk about it. They gained insight about the vulnerability that patients feel in ways that would never have occurred otherwise.

The University of Connecticut School of Medicine has a program called Beginning to End. During their fourth year of medical school, all students are assigned to shadow a patient from the time of admission until discharge. The student's assignment is to record every instance where care could be improved—from lack of professional behavior, communication issues, and housekeeping to waiting times for procedures and tests, nurse response times, and medication errors. Students gain understanding of the workings of a hospital and insights about improving patient care that remain with them throughout their careers. It is a wonderful program. It reinforces, for the student, the importance of the patient as priority one. It identifies opportunities for improvement that are shared with the hospital administration and the faculty of the medical school. It shows the patient that the hospital and school are serious about quality and efficiency of care. Every medical school and teaching hospital should have such a program.

Questions:

1. *Have you ever been hospitalized? If so, what was your experience? Did you feel vulnerable as a patient?*
2. *Remembering your hospital experience, what could have been improved upon?*
3. *If you observe a problem in quality of care involving one of your patients, what do you do about it?*

CHAPTER 7

Innovation

Since we live in an age of innovation, a practical education must prepare a man for work that does not yet exist and cannot yet be clearly defined.

PETER DRUCKER

One evening in 1962, during my second year as a resident at the Massachusetts General Hospital (MGH), I was preparing the discharge sheet for one of the patients on my ward. He had had an uncomplicated heart attack and had completed his four weeks of bed rest in the hospital, the standard treatment of the day. When I went to the patient's bedside to obtain some information from him, he seemed unusually quiet. I asked whether there was something bothering him. He responded that his wife was sexually obsessed, that his recent heart attack had occurred during sex, that once he returned home she would immediately want to resume sex, and that he was afraid to go home for fear of another heart attack. I mouthed some inane words of support and, the next morning, escorted him to the front door of the hospital.

Three weeks later, I received a call from the emergency room—my patient was back with another heart attack. When I went to see him, he looked at me and said, "I told you so." He was transferred back up to the ward and seemed to be convalescing well until one evening he suddenly became unresponsive. I happened to be in his room at the time. Bedside monitors had not yet been developed and obtaining an EKG would have consumed too much time. There was no response to a few thumps on the sternum. I assumed that the patient was in ventricular fibrillation.

I had the ward nurse quickly obtain two long lumbar puncture needles while I stripped the wires from his bedside radio. After attaching the wires to the needles, I inserted one deeply into the right chest and the other into the heart through the left chest. Then I had the nurse repeatedly insert the radio plug into the wall. The whole procedure from his collapse to the external shocking took less than a minute. To our relief, a heartbeat was felt and he awoke. For the next few days, the patient convalesced uneventfully, but, sadly, he was found dead in bed a few days later. I had great difficulty explaining to the patient's wife how it came to be that the power cord on his radio had been stripped.

This episode remains part of the lore of medicine at the MGH, at least among the house officers of the day. But consider the ethical implications of this ad hoc, almost reflex approach to the treatment of an otherwise fatal disturbance of the heart rhythm. The treatment approach had no prior precedent. No informed consent had been possible. Might I have been accused of assaulting the patient?

Experts in the treatment of cardiac arrhythmias would say that a 120-volt shock, even when administered directly to the heart muscle, is not sufficient to reverse ventricular fibrillation. Is it possible that this patient did not have this otherwise fatal arrhythmia?

We tend to forget how much of the medical technology of today is relatively recent. In 1962, coronary angiography and bypass surgery had not yet been developed. External cardiac defibrillators did not exist until 1964. Prior to that time, it was not possible to reverse life-threatening rhythm disturbances such as ventricular tachycardia (or life-ending ventricular fibrillation) except by surgically opening the chest and applying a shock directly to the heart. The few patients finding themselves in this circumstance would be those whose rhythm disturbance occurred in an emergency room (for the evaluation and treatment of a heart attack), where a surgeon would be present and available to open the chest.

Just such a circumstance occurred a few months later when I was on the emergency room rotation. A gentleman was transported to the emergency room by ambulance after suffering an apparent heart attack at work. An EKG showed that he had suffered a massive coronary occlusion. Within minutes, his heart stopped. For all intents and purposes, he was dead. We immediately wheeled him to one of the emergency operating rooms, and the surgical chief resident opened the chest through a rib incision and began to squeeze the heart. Within moments, the patient awoke, climbed off the OR table, and began to walk out of the room, the resident's hand still inside the chest. After a few steps, the patient wrenched free of the resident. He took a few more steps before collapsing on the floor, unconscious. We were unable to get the heart started again, and the poor man was pronounced dead. The entire sequence, from the onset of cardiac arrest till his death, lasted no more than three minutes. Fortunately, I witnessed only a few such horrors in my career.

This could have been an Edgar Allan Poe story. Gratefully, this patient could not have been fully aware of the ghoulish end to his life. His rush from the operating table was most likely a reflex response to the invasion of his body. What remarkable progress has been made in the treatment of cardiac electrical abnormalities since that day! Closed chest massage for cardiac arrest was described two years later. Pacemakers to control rhythm and rate, implantable cardiac defibrillators to prevent death from ventricular fibrillation, and surgical ablation of regions of the heart that induce recurrent abnormalities of heart rhythm followed in subsequent years.

Questions:

1. *What are the basics of cardiac resuscitation? Where does mouth-to-mouth breathing fit in?*
2. *Recall a clinical experience or two that you've had that was gruesome. How did you feel about it?*

CHAPTER 8

Confidentiality

Only one rule in medical ethics need concern you—that action on your part which best conserves the interest of your patient.

MARTIN FISCHER

Physicians at Andrews Air Force Base pulled MOD (medical officer of the day), a twenty-four-hour shift, about once a month. During the day, instead of a schedule of one's own patients, the MOD was responsible for examining and treating patients who just walked in to be seen. Then, from five in the evening until eight the next morning, the MOD saw all adult patients in the emergency room. Children were managed by pediatricians only.

One morning while I was MOD, a senior NCO presented with complaints of abdominal pain. He was a crew chief for Air Force One, the president's plane. As I prepared to examine the patient, I detected alcohol on his breath. The abdominal examination showed that he had an enlarged, slightly tender liver. He also had a few "spiders" on his face and upper chest, red lines radiating out a few millimeters from a small red dot. Almost certainly this was a case of alcoholic liver disease.

I indicated to the patient that his liver was enlarged and tender. I commented about the odor of alcohol on his breath. I indicated that the two were almost certainly connected and that continued drinking would risk his life. I suggested that he seek help through Alcoholics Anonymous. He immediately denied the problem and would entertain no further discussion of the issue.

Here was a conundrum. The patient was not sufficiently ill as to warrant removing him from his position on medical grounds. Yet he was in a role that called for alertness and good judgment. Anything short of this could risk the life of the president. Physicians are expected to maintain the confidentiality of their patient findings. If I shared my findings with his superior, I would be breaching that confidentiality. In the end, my concern for the safety of the president, his staff, and the flight crew of Air Force One carried the day. I informed his commander of my findings and offered suggestions for treatment. The patient was immediately removed from duty and offered the option of treatment or discharge from the air force. He opted for treatment. I never knew whether he succeeded in becoming sober.

Questions:

1. *Was it unethical for me to breach the confidentiality of the doctor-patient interaction?*
2. *By informing his superior, I forced the patient to confront his problem. Was that sufficient justification for breaching confidentiality?*
3. *Should I have talked with his wife first before considering contacting his superior?*
4. *Should I have informed the patient that I would be violating the confidentiality of our relationship by talking with his superior?*
5. *Did the patient's illness really represent a threat to the president and the other passengers and crew of Air Force One? I subsequently found out that the role of crew chief for Air Force One is to oversee those on the ground who maintain the ships. He (or she) does not go up in the plane. Does this role reduce the perceived risk to the president?*

CHAPTER 9

Internship Hours

Fortitude is the marshal of thought, the armor of the will, and the fort of reason

FRANCIS BACON

During my first two years of residency, our on-call schedule averaged about one hundred fifteen hours per week. One week of five nights out of seven alternated with one week of just two of seven. The most grueling part was the Saturday morning to Monday evening on-call stint. I could get through Sunday without any sleep on Saturday night, but if I had had no sleep by Monday, I would have to take a Dexedrine tablet to stay awake the rest of the day. At the time, I thought I was learning so much more than residents with much softer on-call schedules. I conveniently repressed the feelings of exhaustion that characterized so much of the time those two years.

I recall one Sunday night, about two in the morning, without sleep since Friday, trying to start an IV in a patient who had had bilateral posterior cerebral strokes. The poor man was blind from his strokes. His blood pressure was falling. For the life of me, I couldn't get a needle into any of his arm veins. I recall throwing all the IV equipment on the floor in frustration and anger. And, most appallingly, I said (to myself), "Please die so I can get some sleep."

There are many studies that show how impaired an individual's performance is following sleep deprivation. One recent study is particularly relevant. It showed that the frequency of cognitive errors increased by 56 percent among residents who had been caring for patients in an intensive care unit for twenty-four hours in succession.[xv] I'm sure that I made errors as the result of lack of sleep. I'll never know how many or how serious they were.

Medical educators cite the importance of continuity of care and the need to become used to seeing patients under stressful conditions (such as sleep deprivation) as justification for long hours on duty. But the public finds this a specious argument. The average person does not want a sleep-deprived physician caring for him or her when circumstances demand a refreshed mind.

In 1985, a young woman, Libby Zion, died unexpectedly at New York/Cornell Medical Center in the early morning hours. She had been admitted the previous evening with rather bizarre symptoms. No diagnosis had been established. Her father was well connected with the New York City mayor. Following her death, her father insisted that a case of criminal negligence be made against the hospital and the interns and residents who had cared for her. He felt that his daughter had died as the result of poor decisions by exhausted interns and residents.

While a grand jury declined to support such a case, it did recommend a commission to examine the issue of resident work hours. Dr. Howard Axelrod, then the New York State commissioner of health, appointed such a commission. It was headed by Dr. Bertram Bell, a zealot for limits on resident work hours. I was a member of the commission. Politics ruled the day. A limit on work hours was predetermined largely by those chosen to be the members of the commission. Bell wanted a sixty-hour per week limit. I held out for ninety. I didn't think that experiences necessary for diagnosis and management of complex diseases could be achieved in sixty hours a week over three years. The commission agreed on an eighty-hour workweek once it became clear that a recommendation of some limit was inevitable.

The commission also recommended that attending (senior) physicians be available to residents at any hour of the day and night and reside no more than twenty minutes from the hospital. This was a significant recommendation, given that Libby Zion's attending physician spoke with the hospital residents by phone but did not come to the hospital to see her. A third important recommendation was that all hospitals in New York state with ten thousand or more visits to their emergency departments have physicians certified in emergency medicine available twenty-four hours a day. This recommendation was a great stimulus for expanded emergency medicine residency programs across the country.

The eighty-hour workweek was subsequently mandated by the Accreditation Committee for Graduate Medical Education (ACGME), but not until 2004. It remains a contentious mandate, largely because of the logistical difficulties encountered in complying with it. Further, many residents in training, and their teachers, feel that the eighty-hour workweek restriction limits the continuity of patient care and lessens the experience residents gain. Others consider that the eighty-hour workweek represents a reasonable balance among competing objectives. The first is protection of the public through care provided by physicians not suffering from exhausting schedules. The second is a work schedule that provides a balance of adequate training time, continuity of patient care, and attention to one's personal life.

Opponents of the eighty-hour work week might reflect on the success of Rochester's Strong Memorial Hospital in achieving a balance among work hours and time for rest and attention to personal needs, a "night float" system, established in 1939 for coverage of patients by first year residents so that their colleagues could leave when their work was done. On many occasions, the work was not "done" until the middle of the night, but at worst these colleagues were able to get a few hours of rest. Senior residents were on call in the hospital as backup, and attending physicians could be present within fifteen to twenty minutes.

Questions:

1. *Imagine you were a surgical resident and the number of surgical procedures you performed during residency was thought to add to your competency as a surgeon. The eighty-hour workweek is about 20–25 percent shorter than it would have been before the ACGME regulation. The number of procedures you performed would decrease accordingly. Given these figures, what is your opinion of the eighty-hour workweek limitation?*
2. *For how many hours without sleep do you think you can continue to function effectively?*

CHAPTER 10

Help Me Go

The good physician treats the disease; the great physician treats the patient who has the disease.

SIR WILLIAM OSLER

Today, as many as 90 percent of patients with Hodgkin's disease are cured. Until the early 1970s, however, most patients with this disease eventually died from their illness, half within five years. Few of today's physicians have had experience with Hodgkin's patients who no longer respond to treatment. It can be a frightening illness.

I recall a patient I had been treating for some years, a middle-aged businessman. As he became resistant to the few chemotherapeutic drugs we had available at the time, he developed pulmonary involvement. Gradually, lung tissue was replaced by Hodgkin's tumors. Fluid accumulated outside the lung and we had to tap into the fluid with large needles to drain it and give the patient some relief from shortness of breath. Ultimately, his breathing came in shorter and shorter gasps. I came to his bedside with a syringe of morphine. Morphine is highly effective in relieving shortness of breath.

My habit, at the time, was to give just enough morphine to relieve pain or difficulty breathing. I would ask the patient to let me know when he or she had achieved relief. I would then withdraw the needle and dispose of the remaining morphine. In this instance, however, once the patient was breathing better, he looked at me, then at the syringe, and just nodded his head. It was clear what he wanted. The relief I had just provided would last for a few hours at most. Soon I would be back doing what I had just done. I administered just a bit more morphine. He looked at me, smiled, then closed his eyes and peacefully slipped away.

I had just broken the promise I'd made as a new physician—a promise never to take a life. I was so anxious to relieve the suffering of this fine man. It happened so quickly. I have never reconciled this conflict. The moment has remained etched in my memory and vision for all of the forty years that have followed.

Many physicians have had one or more similar experiences. Like me, all would have remained quiet about their intervention. In 1995, an anonymous survey of physicians in the state of Washington found that one in four physicians had received at least one request to help a patient die, and two-thirds had granted such a request.[xvi] The figures were even higher among physicians who treated patients with AIDS (in the days before effective medications to control the disease) and patients with progressive motor weakness, such as amyotrophic lateral sclerosis.

Requests for assistance in dying are not limited to physicians. In a study of critical care nurses, it was found that almost one in five had received at least one request from a patient to hasten death, and one in nine had done so, half without the knowledge of the patient's physician.[xvii] Reducing or discontinuing oxygen, giving more pain medication than is ordered, and letting the drip rate of an intravenous line speed up are among the subtle approaches that can hasten the death of a patient.

In 1986, Dr. Timothy Quill, a practicing internist in Rochester, New York, had the courage to acknowledge in the medical literature that he had assisted in the death of more than one terminally ill patient to relieve intractable suffering. Initially, he was vilified throughout the medical profession. As more and more physicians came forth to share similar stories, the tide of opinion changed. Quill regained the respect of his peers. He is now a much sought-after lecturer on the subject.

Questions:

1. *Have you ever had a patient ask you to help him or her die?*
2. *Have you ever discussed the issue of assisted suicide with your colleagues or teachers?*
3. *How would a member of your family feel about this issue?*
4. *Would you view any treatment that hastens death as going against the Hippocratic oath?*
5. *If you were a terminally ill patient, suffering greatly, what would you ask of your physician?*

CHAPTER 11

Mutiny

The more ignorant, reckless and thoughtless a doctor is, the higher his reputation soars even amongst powerful princes.

DESIDERIUS ERASMUS

We were ten specialists in internal medicine at an Air Force hospital. The chief of medicine was one of them, a nephrologist. We found it impossible to work with him. He was dishonest, lazy, and a poor physician. Most of the rest of us had come from residency and fellowship training programs of the highest quality. And we had all entered the service through the Berry Plan, a program that allowed young physicians to defer their draft obligation until they had completed their training. We were all two-year people. While we were committed to meet our draft obligation, all of us intended to return to civilian life.

As our first year proceeded, my colleagues and I became increasingly concerned about the deficiencies of our chief. His practice of medicine was so poor that patient safety became a paramount concern. He was often absent and we had to see the patients that were scheduled for him in addition to our own. Finally, one Saturday morning, we got together and agreed that we could not, in good conscience, continue to work with this man. In the armed forces, to proceed with such a position against one's commanding officer is recognized as a violation of the Uniform Code of Military Justice, warranting an Article 15, a procedure usually leading to a nonjudicial punishment such as a reduction in rank. We were very much aware of this. But we also knew that our position was based on our concern that this man was incompetent and should not be taking care of patients.

Over the next few weeks, we were careful to document episodes of poor care, unscheduled absences, and lack of professionalism. We took our case to the hospital commander, a physician, a full colonel and a fine man. He listened, respected our concerns, and accepted our documentations of the chief's deficiencies. He did not challenge us for the position we were taking, nor did he indicate what his next steps, if any, would be. We went about our work.

Some two months later, we were informed that our chief was being transferred to a small Air Force hospital in England. We were both pleased and dismayed. While our concerns had been addressed, the problem had simply been transferred to another location. The staff at the hospital in England would be faced with the same issues we had been dealing with. The chief was replaced by an excellent general internist and good manager with whom we enjoyed working for the remainder of our tour of duty.

Three years later, my wife and I were in London on a whirlwind trip. We were enjoying dinner at a quiet restaurant when I looked up and saw the face of the Air Force physician we had had replaced. He was eating dinner alone. Our eyes met and he rose, came over to our table, and greeted us warmly. He indicated that he was no longer seeing patients but, as a career Air Force officer, was happy in his administrative work. We chatted for a while and then he left. Later that evening, as my wife and I were reflecting on this brief interlude, I concluded that two good things had come from his transfer. One was that he was no longer seeing patients. The other was that he appeared to have gained some insight into his weaknesses. I slept better that night.

The armed forces have come a long way since World War II and the Korean War in allowing soldiers to state their case for the removal of an incompetent leader. I would hope that today officers who risk harm to their colleagues or servicemen under them would be relieved of their responsibilities, not just transferred laterally to another command.

Questions:

1. *These issues obviously surface in civilian life as well. Under what circumstances would you feel justified in going over your supervisor's head?*
2. *How might your answer be influenced by concern about being retaliated against as a whistle-blower? Would you worry that your future internship might be jeopardized?*

CHAPTER 12

A Remarkable Response

Synergy and serendipity often play a big part in medical and scientific advances.

JULIE BISHOP

In the spring of 1963, one of my patients being treated for a non-Hodgkin's lymphoma developed an unusual manifestation of the disease. The malignant cells began to escape from capillaries and migrated into the soft tissues under the skin. Within a matter of days, she had developed hundreds of bluish tumors beneath the skin over her entire body. They varied in size from cherries to small plums. At just this time, a new chemotherapeutic drug became available, vinblastine, which was extracted from a common plant, the periwinkle. For hundreds of years, natives of the Caribbean islands had used the leaves of this plant to heal leg ulcers. A pharmaceutical company investigated the healing powers of the plant and found two compounds that appeared to be effective against some tumors (vinblastine and vincristine). Hodgkin's and non-Hodgkin's were among the tumors inhibited by these compounds

I was able to obtain some vinblastine. I prescribed the first dose of the drug and left for a long weekend to attend the wedding of a close friend. When I returned to the patient's bedside on a Monday morning, three days after leaving, I was astounded and excited to see that the hundreds of tumors were rapidly disappearing. Within a few days, they were gone! I had never observed such a rapid response to any chemotherapy. Obviously, the patient was equally ecstatic. She knew her disease was incurable but this reprieve resulted in quite a few months of good health. Subsequently, I had the great good fortune to have many patients who responded well to these drugs. Even today, they remain in the front line of chemotherapy for many tumors.

Question:

1. *Name some other naturally occurring substances that have an important place in medical therapeutics.*

CHAPTER 13

Babies, Babies, Babies

Have a hand in your own treatment. I have nothing but praise for our doctors but I think they could help us better, and we can help them, if we work together.

MARY ANN MOBLEY

During my fourth year in medical school, I was assigned to the obstetrics service over the Christmas holidays. Some of the residents and nurses on the service had taken vacation time. One evening, the obstetrics resident and I delivered twenty-five babies between 5:00 p.m. and 8:00 a.m., a record at the time. There were so many deliveries that each of us was working independently. After delivering a healthy baby from one woman who had twelve other children, I was surprised to see another child's head appear. This twin was delivered easily. In those days (1958), ultrasound had not yet been developed. Unless one heard two heartbeats, twin births were unexpected.

Tied up as I was with this patient, I didn't have time to check on a young woman in the labor room. She was ready to deliver sooner than I was available. Since neither I nor a nurse were around when the time was right, she simply got out of bed, squatted on the floor, and delivered a healthy baby without assistance.

Questions:

2. *What is your reaction to this patient having to deliver her baby without assistance?*
3. *What might have been done to avoid this outcome?*

A few years later, during my time as a hematologist in the air force (and still before ultrasound), a laboratory technician at Walter Reed Medical Center in Washington, DC, developed a technique for predicting the sex of the fetus. He noted that in the third trimester, women who were to deliver a female child had a small percentage of white cells that exhibited a dumbbell shaped attachment to the cell nucleus. This was the extra X chromosome, the other being retained within the body of the nucleus. These white cells were fetal blood cells, cells that had escaped from the fetal circulation, migrated through the placenta, and thence to the mother's circulation. He was correct about 97 percent of the time. Back then, most couples did not want to know the sex of their baby, so his technique was never publicized.

CHAPTER 14

The Giant Spleen

The fact that your patient gets well does not prove that your diagnosis was correct.

SAMUEL J. MELTZER

In 1961, I assumed the care of a patient who had an uncommon blood condition known as myeloid metaplasia (myelofibrosis). This is a clonal disorder of the blood cell precursors in the bone marrow. In most patients, the bone marrow becomes replaced with fibrous tissue, the result of growth factors abnormally released from platelet precursors. At the time, the disease was fatal. While less than half the patients were still alive five years after diagnosis, some lived comfortably for twice as long.

In this disorder, the fibrous tissue infiltration of the marrow interrupts the normal membrane barrier between blood cell growth areas and the capillaries of the marrow. The result is entrance into the blood of immature red and white cells and platelets that accumulate in the spleen (and other organs that capture immature blood cells, such as the liver and lymph nodes). The combination of impaired production of red blood cells and their shortened survival in the circulation results in severe anemia. In most patients, the spleen becomes enlarged as the result of engorgement of immature blood cells.

My patient was a physical therapist, a single woman in her forties who was making the air force her career. Her illness occurred well before bone marrow transplantation had been developed. She had a hugely enlarged spleen, perhaps twenty times its normal size. We now know that an essential function of the spleen is to cleanse the blood of debris, a so-called reticulo-endothelial function. Such debris includes immature blood cells, cells that are less pliant than their mature counterparts. When these cells circulate through the tiny capillaries of the spleen, many are unable to deform well enough to squeeze through the narrow channels. They pile up and, eventually, the spleen enlarges from engorgement with these immature blood cells. Ultimately, the number of cells exceeds the capacity of the spleen to filter them, and other organs with a less efficient filtering function begin to enlarge as well. The liver is one such organ. My patient's liver was enlarged as well as her spleen.

Immature red blood cells are still functioning cells. So in patients with myeloid metaplasia, when their immature red cells become trapped in organs such as the spleen, anemia worsens. This was the case with my patient. Indeed, over the course of her disease, she developed the need for blood transfusions, ultimately requiring as much as two to three units every ten to fourteen days.

The conventional wisdom at the time was that the spleen was enlarged in myeloid metaplasia because it was taking over a function that was failing in the bone marrow—the production of blood cells. This dogma resulted from the observation of pathologists, upon microscopic examination, that blood cells were present in the spleen. Some hematologists, including myself, became convinced that quite the opposite was the case—that the spleen was exerting a destructive influence on circulating blood cells. Published studies of a few hematologists suggested this to be the case from their work on deformability of immature blood cells.

I suggested that we remove the patient's spleen, speculating that by removing an organ that was destroying young blood cells, the patient's extraordinary requirements for blood transfusions would be reduced. Our pathologists insisted that such treatment would be disastrous, that it would eliminate an organ that was attempting to make up for what the bone marrow was lacking. Given the conflicting opinions, we submitted the case to a peer group of hematologists and pathologists. They agreed with my proposed approach.

I then sat with the patient and explained the reasoning for my proposal that her spleen be removed. We discussed the possible outcomes. She was so tired of having to be transfused so often that she accepted the risk. We proceeded to remove her spleen. Her postoperative convalescence was uneventful. As we had hoped, her need for transfusions fell dramatically. From two units of blood every ten to fourteen days, she now required transfusions only every three to four months. She was ecstatic. We had confirmed that the spleen was indeed destructive, not productive, in myeloid metaplasia.

The patient continued to do well, so I was shocked to learn, after returning from a weekend out of town, that she had died suddenly the previous Saturday. She had gone to the emergency room of the hospital with a slight fever and cough. She received a prescription for penicillin, but before she'd even had it filled, she'd collapsed and died. At autopsy, her bloodstream was found to be filled with pneumococcal organisms, the most common cause of pneumonia.

The spleen is an effective filter of such organisms. Without it, she was not able to contain the infection. Some years after she died, a vaccine to prevent pneumococcal infection was developed (Pneumovax). Had it been available at the time of her splenectomy, she would have received the vaccine. Pneumovax is now routinely given to all patients whose spleen has been removed. Her untimely death notwithstanding, this patient benefited greatly from her splenectomy, enjoying a good quality of life despite her serious bone marrow disorder.

Today, allogeneic bone marrow transplantation may be curative in patients with myelofibrosis. Younger patients do better than older, and transplantation is usually recommended when poor prognostic signs, such as severe anemia, become more prominent.

Disagreements are common in medical practice. Most are in circumstances where there is little or no information about the "right" course. Patients are participating more and more in decisions relating to their care, particularly when it is not known whether one type of treatment is better than another—so-called shared decision-making.[xviii] Treatment of patients with cancer of the prostate is one such example where the patient's values and preferences regarding differing complications are important determinants.

Questions:

1. *What are some of the things that one should not do when disagreements occur between physicians about diagnosis or treatment?*
2. *What information sources might you use to help resolve conflicts of opinion?*
3. *How should one approach the patient when such differences occur?*

CHAPTER 15

Legionnaires' Disease

Bedside manners are no substitute for the right diagnosis

ALFRED P. SLOAN

I was called to see a forty-three-year-old white male at one of our local community hospitals. He had gone out for a golf game with three of his friends, and when he hit his tee shot, he experienced sudden, severe, sharp pain in the sternal area. The pain abated somewhat as he walked to his golf ball. He decided to hit his second shot. It was a fine shot, landing on the green three feet from the cup. This golf swing, however, was immediately followed by a recurrence of the same severe chest pain. He was able to walk to the green and sink his putt for a birdie but then left and drove to the emergency room of the community hospital.

Physical examination revealed an exquisitely tender sternum, but there were no other physical findings. An EKG was normal and he was then sent for a chest x-ray, which showed a fractured sternum and multiple healing rib fractures. The radiologist commented on a striking loss of density throughout all his bone structures. He was hospitalized for further study. Blood tests revealed extraordinary increases in blood calcium (18mg/dl) and total protein (14gm/dl).

The elevated protein level was studied further and shown to be composed mostly of a monoclonal gamma globulin. A bone marrow examination showed that about 60 percent of his bone marrow cells consisted of plasma cells. Normal levels would be 0.5–1.5 percent. These cells produce a protein that has a characteristic pattern when blood is subjected to protein analysis. Plasma cells leach calcium from bone, thus explaining the x-ray finding of the loss of bone density and the very high calcium level. The findings confirmed the diagnosis of multiple myeloma, a bone marrow malignancy represented by an abnormal clone of plasma cells.

When I first saw and examined this patient, he indicated that he had had some pains in his back and chest over the past year when playing football with his sons. When further bone x-rays were obtained, compression fractures of two lumbar vertebrae were found. I was amazed by the patient's tolerance for pain. It was clear that the signs of his multiple myeloma had been present for more than a year and that his body had slowly adapted to the rising protein and calcium levels in his blood that would otherwise have been lethal.

This patient's illness occurred prior to the era of bone marrow transplantation. At the time, it was uniformly fatal. Most patients responded well to chemotherapy that was quite easy to tolerate, a single tablet taken on a daily basis. Survivals of six to nine years were recorded. Today, the patient would likely have opted for a bone marrow transplant; when successful, it is curative.

Indeed, the patient's disease was highly responsive to chemotherapy. Within a matter of weeks, his bone pains disappeared. The high calcium level, a risk to his kidney function, was brought down to safe levels with appropriate medication. The abnormal protein disappeared from the blood within about three months, and, in parallel, the bone marrow reverted to normal. He had a new lease on life. He returned to his habit of playing football with his sons, a practice that I did not support. It was, however, a telling indication of his return to normal health.

The patient remained in good health for about five years. As a salesman, he was frequently on the road. He tolerated his trips well until he returned from a convention in Phoenix, Arizona, with a "cold." A few days later, fever, chills, and cough ensued and he contacted me. When he was seen in our emergency room, he was obviously ill, with a temperature of 103 degrees and rales on examination of the lungs suggestive of pneumonia. A chest x-ray confirmed the suspicion.

He was admitted to the hospital and placed on a broad-spectrum antibiotic. While there was no evidence of recurrence of his multiple myeloma, he remained acutely ill and was transferred to the intensive care unit. Cultures of sputum and blood were negative. Despite close medical attention, he deteriorated rapidly and died within a few days. I was almost as distressed as his wife and sons. To lose him after such a remarkable response to treatment was difficult.

The patient's death occurred at about the time that Legionnaires' disease was first described (1976) following an outbreak of pneumonia at an American Legion convention in Philadelphia. Legionnaires' disease is an illness due to a bacterium, *Legionella* species, found in the water supply of air conditioning units and identified as the culprit responsible for outbreaks of acute respiratory infections among people attending conventions and other meetings in close quarters. Postmortem cultures of the lungs of my patient revealed *Legionella*, the first case recognized in upstate New York.

I was dismayed. Shouldn't I have suspected the disease given that he had been to a convention, the venue where the earliest cases of Legionnaires' disease had been described? That his compromised immune system may have precluded his survival in any case and that the antibiotics available to treat the disease were only modestly successful did not excuse the failure to consider the diagnosis of Legionnaires'.

Question:

1. *Remember* primum non nocere. *Does this story indicate that harm was done to the patient through an error of omission; that is, not considering Legionnaires' disease as the cause of the patient's pneumonia?*

CHAPTER 16

The General's Mother

Science is the father of knowledge but opinion breeds ignorance.

HIPPOCRATES

I was asked to see a pleasant elderly woman, the mother of a general. The patient said that she was concerned about an increase in the girth of her abdomen. She noted that her waist size had increased two inches over the past two months without any increase in body weight. There had been no abdominal symptoms. Indeed, she had no symptoms of any kind other than the increase in size of her abdomen. Her abdomen was somewhat protuberant but did not appear distended. It was not tender. No organs or masses could be detected.

What could result in such an increase in the size of her abdomen without any evidence of a mass? Might it be fluid? I checked the location on the right side of the abdomen where the percussion note was dull, where the lateral abdominal wall was lower than the level of the bowel and thus where a percussion note no longer sounded like a drum. Then I turned the patient partly on her side and checked the point of dullness again. It was at least one inch above the original point, a sure sign of fluid within the abdomen.

I informed the patient that her increase in abdominal girth was most likely due to the accumulation of fluid in the abdominal cavity. I suggested that an abdominal tap was indicated to confirm the presence of fluid and examine its cause by submitting the fluid to microscopic evaluation. Hospitalization was arranged, with plans to tap the abdomen the following morning.

The patient's daughter-in-law alerted her husband, an air force general, about my preliminary diagnosis and plan to tap the abdomen for fluid. He suggested an independent evaluation, and the hospital commander arranged for a gastroenterologist from one of the medical schools in Washington to see the patient that evening. Confident in my diagnosis, I was entirely supportive of this consultation. But the gastroenterologist disagreed with my findings, suggesting, in what I felt was a condescending manner, that her abdominal protuberance was simply a manifestation of diastasis recti. That term is used to describe the separation of the abdominal rectus muscles from the midline of the abdomen, leaving the central portion of the abdomen soft to touch.

How could diastasis recti explain a two-inch increase in abdominal girth? I asked myself. I was confident that the increase was due to the accumulation of fluid, so I made arrangements for an abdominal tap first thing in the morning.

The next morning, at the patient's bedside, the head nurse said, "You know what will happen if you don't find fluid, don't you?" he asked, implying a court martial. I said, "Not to worry." After administering a local anesthetic, I entered the abdominal cavity with the cannula, immediately noting the flow of slightly cloudy, yellow fluid. Two gallons were removed, more than enough to explain her increase in abdominal girth!

Microscopic examination of the fluid revealed malignant "signet rings," cells typical of ovarian cancer. The patient was distressed, of course, after learning about the cause of her abdominal swelling but grateful that I had listened to her and believed her. She accepted treatment with chemotherapy and enjoyed a comfortable life for some months afterward.

The patient's physician is not obligated to accept the opinion of a consultant. However, if he or she does not, the reason should be clearly stated in the medical record and reviewed with the patient.

Questions:

1. *There was a clue from the medical history that suggested the possibility of fluid in the abdomen. What was it?*
2. *What other diseases can cause fluid to accumulate in the abdominal cavity?*
3. *How does the color of intra-abdominal fluid influence the diagnosis of its cause?*

CHAPTER 17

Life-Changing Treatment

Diagnosis is not the end but the beginning of practice.

MARTIN H. FISCHER

In the late 1960s, I was referred a young adult male for evaluation of anemia. His wife accompanied him to the examining room. She provided most of the history since he was a bit lethargic and slow of speech. She indicated that he had been quiet and reserved since she first met him, but that over the past year, sleepiness had become a serious problem—he was becoming mentally sluggish and less interested in sex. His snoring at night was becoming more pronounced, and he frequently slept past his alarm, losing time from work.

Abnormal findings on physical examination included a slow pulse, a slightly puffy appearance to his face, and markedly delayed relaxation of his deep tendon reflexes. Almost certainly, he had severe hypothyroidism. A blood test of thyroid function showed that the level of thyroxin (T4), the principal thyroid hormone, was almost zero, confirming the diagnosis. Anemia, the reason he was referred to me, is common in patients with hypothyroidism. Most often, the low red cell counts return to normal after thyroid replacement therapy.

Hypothyroidism is much less common in males than females, particularly in younger people. This is probably because primary hypothyroidism is most frequently the result of an autoimmune process (thyroiditis) that destroys thyroid tissue and the ability to produce thyroid hormone. This process is far more frequent in women than men. Conversely, various disturbances of the pituitary gland or the hypothalamus section of the brain may result in a decrease in the neuro-humoral "signal" that stimulates the thyroid to produce thyroid hormone. This signal is thyroid-stimulating hormone (TSH), produced by the pituitary, and results in the thyroid gland ultimately producing the active hormones thyroxin and triiodothyronine. These disturbances may be congenital or acquired (i.e. tumors, infection). Often the cause is unknown.

Interestingly, obstructive sleep apnea is a well-recognized consequence of hypothyroidism, and we postulated that the patient's daytime sleepiness and loud snoring at night were probably manifestations of this complication.

At the time this patient was seen, commercial techniques did not exist to measure the production of TSH or the presence of thyroid antibodies. We will never know whether the patient's underactive thyroid was due to decreased central (e.g., brain) stimulation (lack of TSH) or was due to a diseased gland (inability to respond to normal pituitary hormonal stimulus). In any case, treatment with thyroid hormone replacement would have been the same.

The patient was referred back to his primary physician with the recommendation that a low dose of thyroid replacement be started and be increased to full replacement levels over a period of three months. We asked to see the patient in six months.

When the patient returned, we noted a dramatic change. He no longer appeared sleepy or dull of speech. Indeed, he was alert, pacing around the examining room and speaking quite rapidly. His wife indicated that he was no longer snoring at night and was always up first thing in the morning. His abnormal physical findings had disappeared and his anemia was corrected. The thyroid hormone levels were later noted to be in the normal range. My resident and I were pleased to see the results of our treatment.

But we were in for quite a shock! The patient's wife said, "He is no longer the quiet, reserved, reliable, uncomplicated man that I fell in love with and married. He's rushing around all the time. He has obtained a second job. He's purchased a motorcycle and rides off with it in the evening. I never see him any more, and I think he is meeting other women." Subsequently, we learned that the marriage had failed.

Here was a man who had probably been hypothyroid for years, certainly for as long as his wife had known him, throughout their courtship and marriage. Most likely, he had been hypothyroid during his adolescent years. Now, suddenly, with normal thyroid hormones circulating, he must have gone through an accelerated adolescence, and his persona was so very different than the man his wife had known and fallen in love with.

Questions:

1. *What have you learned from this patient story?*
2. *Can you think of any other diseases that should be treated slowly to avoid adverse consequences of treatment?*

CHAPTER 18

The Difficult Patient

A man that studieth revenge keeps his own wounds green.

FRANCIS BACON

One of my patients with acute leukemia was admitted to the hospital late one evening in the fall of 1967. He was a gentleman who felt that life had not treated him fairly. His wife and daughter indicated that he was a person who was always waiting for something good to come to him rather than seeking opportunity himself. He had become a rather bitter, angry man.

Well, the only bed left in the hospital was the largest of all the private rooms. And did my patient relish this gift! He began to act as lord of the manor, giving orders to staff and being generally obnoxious. Early one evening, as the intern assigned to him walked by the door, the patient called out for him to come in. The intern looked in the door and said that his colleague would be in as soon as possible. The patient made short shrift of the colleague, complaining about the fact that his intern had abandoned him.

The next morning, when the intern walked into the room, the patient exploded. He said, "Mr. Smith—I'll not call you *Doctor* Smith because you don't deserve it—you abandoned me last evening. In my opinion, you are so small that you could walk under a duck with a top hat on and not ruffle its feathers. You're fired!" Wow! The patient must have been ruminating all night about what he was going to say to the intern.

A few moments later, I ran into the intern. He was hurt and confused. The evening before, after being on duty for thirty-six hours straight, he was leaving the ward to return to his quarters for a meal and some rest when the patient spied him walking past the door. He felt he had been unfairly treated by the patient. I agreed with the intern but suggested that it would have been more diplomatic if he had indicated to the patient that he was off duty and quite exhausted before telling him that his colleague would be in to see him.

We walked back into the patient's room together, and I explained to the patient what the intern had just shared with me, that he had been exhausted and felt that his colleague could handle the patient's request. I suggested to the patient that, having fired his intern, he (the patient) had two options. One was to apologize to the intern; the other was for me to arrange his transfer to an affiliated hospital where a colleague of mine would be pleased to accept him as a patient. The patient immediately apologized to the intern. He and the intern subsequently became fast friends.

It is almost always possible for physicians to learn ways to manage difficult patients if they understand them. Sir William Osler wrote, "It is much more important to know what sort of a patient has a disease than what sort of a disease a patient has."

Difficult patients often express their anxiety through anger, challenging the medical establishment in ways that may be trying. It's always gratifying when the medical or nursing staff succeed in meeting the needs of the difficult patient.

Not all difficult encounters are due to the patient. Stress, physical exhaustion, and sleep deprivation can result in the physician being less caring or finding it difficult to manage a complex patient.

Questions:

3. *Have you encountered a difficult patient or family? If so, how did you handle it? Were you satisfied with the outcome?*
4. *What approaches would you take with* all *patients to help ensure a good relationship?*

CHAPTER 19

The Power over Life

Whenever a doctor cannot do good, he must be kept from doing harm.

HIPPOCRATES

When I was a resident in medicine, one of my interns was a bright young man who was also brash and flippant. One afternoon, he received a patient from the emergency room with a severe penicillin reaction. When the patient had arrived, he had been gasping for breath and had a generalized, itchy rash. He responded well to treatment, but the reaction was sufficiently serious that hospitalization was felt advisable to monitor his progress.

After the intern took a history and completed a physical examination, he walked by the nursing station and said to the nurse, "Six hundred thousand units of aqueous penicillin." At that time, many medications were kept in a closet in the nurses' station instead of in the central pharmacy.

Penicillin was one such medication. The nurse proceeded to fill a syringe with six hundred thousand units of penicillin, went to the patient's bedside, and administered it to him. No more than fifteen seconds later, he suddenly asked, "My God, what did you give me, penicillin?" He gasped a few times and died.

How easy it is to take a patient's life, and how easy it is to destroy one's career. Both the intern and the nurse lost their jobs. The intern finished his training at a mediocre hospital and went into practice in a remote community in Texas. The nurse eventually secured a position at a rural hospital in Nebraska. What the intern should never have said is obvious. What the nurse should not have done was to act on a verbal order. Asking the intern to write out what he had asked her to do would have prevented the tragedy. Nurses were not allowed to accept verbal orders except in life-threatening situations.

The patient's family sued the hospital, the employer of both the intern and the nurse. The suit was settled for a figure far lower than the amount that was sought because the sixty-five-year old patient with a calculated life expectancy of only twelve years had "limited value." I've always felt that such terms are demeaning. The patient's value to his family was inestimable.

I use this sad story with all new medical students and interns. It is a tragic example of how much power the physician has over life and how important it is to hold that power in great respect. There is no room for thoughtless acts in the practice of medicine.

Questions:

1. *Have you ever observed a silly act by a physician that could have caused serious harm to a patient? What was your reaction?*
2. *What is the preferred treatment for an acute allergic reaction such as a penicillin reaction?*
3. *What should a patient with a severe food allergy always have available for the immediate treatment of an allergic reaction?*

CHAPTER 20

Arrogance

There are only two sorts of doctors: those who practice with their brains and those who practice with their tongues.

SIR WILLIAM OSLER

One day during my internship, I sent a patient next door to the Massachusetts Eye and Ear Infirmary to obtain a bronchoscopy. A chest x-ray had shown what appeared to be a tumor pressing upon and possibly invading the left main bronchus. A bronchoscope is an instrument with a reflecting mirror that permits one to view the bronchial passages. If necessary, a smaller instrument can be inserted through the scope to biopsy or cauterize tissue. Today's bronchoscopes are flexible fiber-optic instruments that are relatively easy to manipulate under trained hands. During my residency, the bronchoscopes were rigid metal instruments. They were more difficult to handle.

The patient underwent the procedure, a biopsy was done, and he was returned to the floor. Within about an hour, he began to develop an amazing amount of air beneath the skin, a condition known as subcutaneous emphysema. In this case, the finding was almost certainly due to a perforation of the bronchus at the time of bronchoscopy. Air leaks out of the bronchus into the chest cavity. It then dissects along fascial planes. The tissues beneath the skin fill with air. The body appears greatly swollen. When one touches a swollen body part, the tissue feels soft and it crackles. This patient's findings were so extreme that his entire scalp was lifted up from the cranium. Surprisingly, he was in no distress.

I called the office of the physician who had done the procedure and spoke with him, describing what I was observing. He replied that he had performed more than ten thousand bronchoscopies without ever having such a complication and that I must be wrong. So I asked, "Sir, what do you suggest I do with this mirage?" That got his attention. He promptly came to see the patient and confirmed the finding. In this case, fortunately, the small hole that must have been created sealed itself spontaneously and the air beneath the skin gradually reabsorbed over a day or two.

Today, subcutaneous emphysema is most commonly seen as a complication of endotracheal intubation. It has also been described after cocaine use, presumably due to thermal injury along the respiratory tract. Subcutaneous emphysema of the back and thighs may result from perforation of the colon during colonoscopy.

Beware of the arrogant physician. He or she is likely to be more interested in self than the patient. Such physicians are less willing to engage patients in decisions about treatment and are more prone to errors. Sadly, only after a preventable event such as an unnecessary death or serious complication may they acquire some humility.

Questions:

1. *Have you worked with an attending physician whose demeanor was arrogant? How did the nursing staff deal with the physician?*
2. *On the fine line between confidence and arrogance, where do you fit?*
3. *Is there any difference in how you deal with criticism when you are wearing the white coat than when you are not? If your answer is yes, explain why.*

CHAPTER 21

Ad Hoc Survey

I like to listen. I have learned a great deal from listening. Most people never listen.

Ernest Hemingway

During my year as chief resident in medicine, I found a unique way of "taking the pulse" of the hospitalized male patients on the medical service. A small men's room was next to my office. A large ventilation shaft connected this men's room with the communal toilets of the male ward. From the men's room, one could hear virtually everything that was said in the toilets. I used to sit and listen to the banter of the men. It gave me a good idea of how they felt about the hospital and the teaching attending physicians.

One morning, I listened to a patient complaining about the fact that he was being examined so often—first by an intern, then the resident, then the attending physician, and then by two different consultants. Why didn't they just read the information obtained by the intern?

Soon, another patient spoke up. He said, "Well, I don't agree with you. I come from a small community fifty miles south of here. My doctor couldn't figure out what was wrong with me, so he sent me up here. Yes, there are many people who examine you. But you know what? After they've all had a go at you, they get together and talk about you. And they all come around the bedside to check and make sure that what they heard from you was correct. They work like a team, and they figured out what was wrong with me. Now I'm on the mend. And I'm thankful. I have to think this is a good way to do things."

From this listening post, I learned what the male patients thought about the hospital and its physicians. Being examined by medical students and multiple physicians can be very tiring indeed. But these multiple observations can result in big payoffs. There are many stories of patients with elusive symptoms and signs whose diagnosis was made by a careful student or intern, not by the senior resident or attending physician.

Question:

1. *Many would say that my observations were an invasion of privacy. Hospitalized patients shouldn't have to be concerned that their words are being surreptitiously monitored.What do you think?*

PART TWO

The Importance of Good Bedside Skills
Listening, Observing, Examining

The stories in this part of the book should convince the reader that no amount of diagnostic testing can substitute for the information that comes from listening, observing, and the laying on of hands. Most diagnoses can be suspected by clues obtained from the patient's history; the story in chapter 23 is a case in point. At times, what the physician observes or feels results in the diagnostic clue, as seen in the story described in chapter 34. When these tasks are performed carefully, both the patient and the physician gain confidence.

CHAPTER 22

Locked In

Patients and their families will forgive you for wrong diagnoses but will rarely forgive you for wrong prognoses; the older you grow in medicine the charier you get about offering ironclad prognoses, good or bad.

ANONYMOUS

In *How Doctors Think,* Dr. Jerome Groopman reflects on the reasoning process that doctors use to arrive at a diagnosis.[xix] He refers to the problem of physicians becoming "locked in" to a diagnosis so early in the process that they overlook the important clues. The result, so often, is an incorrect diagnosis and inappropriate treatment.

The best example I can recall involved a close friend. He had developed a chronic pain in the right hip and was referred to an orthopedic surgeon for advice. The surgeon obtained a CT scan of the hip. It showed some activity at the head of the femur, suggesting the possibility of a cancerous growth. The friend was notified and he called me for advice. I suggested he arrange a visit with an oncologist at the university hospital located in his hometown. I flew up to be with him during a day of consultations and examinations.

The first visit to the oncologist set the tone for the day. It was assumed that he had a malignancy involving the head of the femur. A CT scan of the hip showed increased blood flow, furthering the conclusion that there was a tumor. I asked whether the pain could be due to aseptic necrosis of the hip. The response was, "Oh, no, the nuclear scan would not light up like this—just the opposite."

A chest x-ray showed multiple tiny spots. I recall seeing such tiny spots on my own chest x-ray of some years ago. The radiologist, equipped with the referral note from the oncologist and the interpretation of the CT scan, said to me, "This has to be metastatic carcinoma." We never asked my friend when and where his last chest x-ray had been taken.

Late in the afternoon, the oncologist called us back in and indicated to my friend that all findings indicated a cancer that had traveled to bone and lung. There are three cancers in men that metastasize to both bone and lung: prostate, lung, and lymphoma. A biopsy of the hip lesion was arranged, and we returned home where the friend sat down with his family and shared what the doctors had said. He indicated that he had had a good life and was ready to die. Many tears were shed.

I was uneasy. The friend looked awfully healthy for a man with a tumor that had metastasized to his lungs and bone. Lo and behold, when the biopsy was done, there was no cancer found. What *was* found was evidence of aseptic necrosis, which was healing spontaneously, thus explaining the findings on the CT scan. There was much cheering and more tears among the family members.

This is a powerful example of how physicians can become blinded to evidence, once having prematurely locked themselves into a diagnosis.

Questions:

1. *Can you recall instances where you have closed out other diagnostic possibilities prematurely? How early in the diagnostic process did this happen?*
2. *What is the most common reason for becoming locked into an incorrect diagnosis?*

CHAPTER 23

The Abnormal EKG

A doctor who cannot take a good history and a patient who cannot give one are in danger of giving and receiving bad treatment.

ANONYMOUS

One of my patients had carried the diagnosis of coronary heart disease with angina for some ten years before I first saw her. On her first visit to me, she indicated that brief episodes of burning substernal pain occurred with regularity, but the discomfort was not related to exertion. She brought her medical record with her. Notes from some of the most respected physicians in Boston accompanied a set of EKGs that I can only describe as scary changes that indicated severe restriction of blood flow to the left ventricle. Indeed, when I showed these EKGs to colleagues, they asked where she was. I replied, "She is in my office." To a person, they said, "She should be in the coronary care unit."

The woman was a patient before the advent of coronary angiography and coronary bypass surgery, so I continued to treat her conservatively with nitroglycerin and rest. Remarkably, she did well for some years until, on one visit; she indicated that the pain was now occurring at night, awakening her from sleep. It was not accompanied by shortness of breath or any other symptoms suggesting heart failure, nor did her heart sounds indicate a sign of failure.

I asked if she was doing anything differently in the evenings. She replied, "Well, my husband and I have a few drinks before retiring." I asked what she was drinking and how much. She replied, "Six Manhattans."

A light suddenly went on, one that should have been on when I first saw her. After exploring her symptoms in more detail, I concluded that her chest pain was due to reflux esophagitis. Could this have been the case all these years? This is indeed what was found. Examination with a gastroscope of her esophagus and stomach revealed multiple severe esophageal ulcers, the result of acid reflux. She was treated with antacids and acid-blocking drugs, and the symptoms disappeared almost immediately.

This is another example of becoming "locked in" on a diagnosis when subsequent events indicate the need to reexamine whether it is indeed correct. The patient suffered needlessly for a number of years because I accepted, without question, that her chest pain was caused by the previously diagnosed coronary heart disease.

A year or two later, the patient came to the emergency room with severe pain in the right upper quadrant of her abdomen. The area was tender to touch but no mass was felt. A gallbladder study (oral cholecystogram) revealed the presence of gallstones. The abdominal pain was felt to be the result of a stone impacting the gallbladder duct. A decision was made to perform a cholecystectomy. Just before the patient was to be called to the operating room, I stopped by to see her one more time. The area of pain now showed a red blistering rash. Shingles!

Surgery was cancelled, instructions were given to the patient about care of the rash, and she was sent home. In time, the rash and pain disappeared. Her gallbladder was never removed.

This experience taught me the importance of repeated observation and examination of the patient when there is any diagnostic uncertainty.

Question:

1. *What is best practice for the treatment of asymptomatic gallstones?*

CHAPTER 24

The Resident's Wife

Get your facts first, then you can distort them as you please.

MARK TWAIN

One afternoon in clinic, one of the residents came to me and asked if I would look at a blood smear. I examined the slide under the microscope. The findings were classic for iron deficiency. The red cells were pale with odd shapes characteristic of iron deficiency. Some were fragmented. The white cells and platelets appeared to be normal.

I asked the resident whether it was his blood smear. No, it was his wife's. Then I asked whether she was running for exercise. He replied that indeed she was. I indicated to him that running can result in damage to red blood cells during their circulation through the foot. The damage is observed on the blood smear as fragments of cells. Iron is then released from the damaged cells and excreted in the urine. Over time, deficiency of iron can occur. This is particularly so in women in the childbearing ages because of the additional iron they lose during their menstrual periods.

Throughout our conversation, he repeatedly asked whether the blood smear could indicate leukemia. Just as repeatedly, I said no. It took all my powers of persuasion to convince the resident that the findings on the blood smear were perfectly benign. He had been so sure that his dear wife had leukemia that he could not hear the reasoning that indicated she was simply deficient in iron.

A final example of becoming locked in. Medical students and physicians in training often focus on the worst of diagnostic possibilities when they or a close family member are ill. Dr. Theodore Woodward, a revered chair of medicine at the University of Maryland in the mid-twentieth century was fond of saying, "When you hear hoof beats behind you, don't think of zebras." Some learners need frequent reminders of this aphorism.

Question:

1. *What are some of the serious diseases you have been convinced you had?*

CHAPTER 25

Yes, Doctor

The doctor may learn more about the illness from the way the patient tells the story than from the story itself.

JAMES B. HERRICK

Every Tuesday, we held "professors' rounds" at the University of Rochester Medical Center. Lawrence Young (the chair of medicine), William Morgan (an associate chair), and I (the other associate chair) each took one-third of the residents and spent two hours discussing a single patient at length. We always began at the bedside. The patients selected for these rounds appreciated the additional attention to their cases. The patient's medical history and physical examination findings were presented in detail. The patients were always impressed with how much information had been obtained from the residents about their illnesses.

On one of these rounds, I asked the patient, an elderly woman, a number of questions. Her yes or no responses were always followed by "doctor."

When we retired to the conference room to discuss the patient, I asked the resident team what the patient's religion was. They replied that her religious affiliation had not been brought up at the bedside. I said that it had not been necessary; her "yes, doctor," "no, doctor" responses indicated that she was Catholic, having been brought up in the Catholic school system where questions of teachers were answered either by "yes, father" or "yes, sister."

This brief anecdote points to the information that can be obtained simply by listening to how the patient responds to questions.

Question:

1. *There are many observations one can make by the bedside that give clues to the patient's beliefs and values. Can you name some?*

CHAPTER 26

Prelude to Suicide

Life's but a walking shadow, a poor player that struts and frets his hour upon the stage and then is heard no more.

WILLIAM SHAKESPEARE

Rheumatoid spondylitis is a chronic and ultimately debilitating disorder of the spine. The anterior longitudinal spinal ligaments become calcified and rigid. As the ligaments contract, the spine bends forward. Ultimately, the patient is hunched over as the cervical and thoracic spine becomes bowed. Pain is less of a problem than the disability caused by the bent spine. These changes take place over many years.

During my time in the air force, one of my patients was a civilian employee at the Pentagon. He had rheumatoid spondylitis and was functioning quite well despite living with the disease for quite some years. We developed a close rapport. I remember arranging for him to have preferred parking at the Pentagon because he had to walk a good quarter of a mile from his car to his office—quite a challenge with his condition.

He and his wife entertained my wife and me on a number of occasions. When I left the air force to return to Boston to complete my training, he was one of the patients I missed the most.

Some five years later, at about nine o'clock one Saturday evening, I received a call at our home in Rochester, New York. It was from this patient. I had not heard from him since leaving the air force. We talked for about half an hour. He indicated that he and his wife were now divorced. His spondylitis was progressing, and it appeared that he would soon have to retire. He regretted that he and his wife had had no children. I responded in as supportive a way as I could. Finally, he said, "Good-bye, Dr. Griner" and hung up the phone. I said to myself, "Oh, my God, he's going to kill himself." I immediately contacted the police in his community. They sped over to his house, only to find him dead from a self-inflicted gunshot wound.

I've often wondered whether I could have picked up on the clue that he was calling the only support person left in his life to say good-bye before taking his life. Had I been more observant, I might have changed the outcome by continuing to talk with him while my wife contacted the police in his locale.

Question:

1. *If I had recognized the suicide intent while the person was on the phone, what might I have done other than to call the police?*

CHAPTER 27

Unexplained Findings

They certainly give very strange and newfangled names to diseases.

PLATO

One day during my fourth year in medical school, I was advised that a patient had been hospitalized on our medical service for about ten days with a high-spiking fever, but no cause had been identified. This was a woman in her late twenties. Her medical history was unremarkable. She indicated that the fever began suddenly with no premonitory symptoms.

There were no abnormal physical findings. Cultures of blood and urine for the presence of bacteria were negative. A large battery of laboratory tests and conventional x-rays had revealed no abnormal findings. This was in the days before modern imaging with CT and MRI and radionuclide scans. Her physicians had pored over the recently published article by McDermott and Petersdorf, "Fever of Unknown Origin."[xx] This paper was a classic in the field. It traced the course of patients with protracted fevers whose causes were unknown (FUO) after extensive study. The authors found that in a significant number of cases, a source in the abdomen—rare tumors, abscesses, and the like—were eventually identified through surgical exploration.

Our patient's temperature readings, obtained via a rectal thermometer, varied from 101 to 105 degrees with no particular regularity. Interestingly, the patient's pulse was normal, and she had no sweats or chills. Most often, a temperature of this level would be accompanied by a rapid pulse. Typhoid fever is an exception, the pulse often being normal or near normal in the face of high fever. However, the negative cultures for bacteria effectively ruled out typhoid.

A surgical consultation was obtained and agreement reached on a decision to explore the abdomen. Before surgery could be scheduled, an observant nurse asked the patient to provide a urine specimen during one of her temperature spikes to 105 degrees. The nurse then measured the temperature of the urine sample and noted that it was 98.4 degrees!

Questions:

1. *How could this be?*
2. *What other findings were highly unusual in this patient?*

This next story is another example of the same disorder.

On another occasion that same year, a young woman came to the clinic with the complaint that her urine was bloody. The problem, she noted, had been present for about two days. Her last menstrual period had been ten days earlier, and she had not had vaginal bleeding since then. She did not have any other symptoms. In particular, there was no pain on urination, fever, or urinary frequency or urgency, and she had not noted this problem in the past.

The patient was given a cup and instructed to provide a urine sample. The sample she provided was pinkish red. A medical student examined the urine specimen under the microscope and found that it contained innumerable red blood cells. But they were huge and they had nuclei! Impossible, we said, as human red cells do not have nuclei. Perhaps he was seeing something else.

We examined the sample ourselves and were stunned to confirm that the student had indeed identified nucleated red blood cells.

Question

1. *How do you explain this finding?*

These two women had factitious disorder, often used interchangeably with Munchausen syndrome, named after an eighteenth century German officer who had a compulsion to embellish stories of his life experiences. This mental illness is observed most often in young women, many of whom have been employed in the health field. They may falsify an illness, as we see in these two cases, or deliberately cause an illness such as injecting themselves with infected material. They often move from hospital to hospital, seeking attention, obtaining unnecessary tests, procedures, and even surgery, such as exploratory laparotomy.

Clues to the diagnosis of factitious disorder come from careful listening and observation. The medical history may be quite dramatic but accompanied by inconsistent or vague details. The patient's knowledge of medical terms and diseases may be greater than expected for someone without training in the health professions. The patient may be eager to undergo uncomfortable tests and procedures. Symptoms may be present only when the patient is being observed. Completely normal findings on physical examination in the face of striking symptoms should lead to the suspicion of factitious disorder, so too should the finding of completely normal diagnostic test results.

The factors responsible for this disorder are not known. Unfortunately, patients most often do not improve after psychiatric treatment.

In the first case described above, there were multiple clues to the diagnosis of factitious disorder. First was the discrepancy between the elevated thermometer readings and the lack of associated physical findings such as sweating, rapid pulse, lethargy, or warm skin. The second clue was that the laboratory values and diagnostic procedures all showed normal results.

Only after many days in the hospital did an observant nurse note the lack of body warmth in the face of an apparent high fever. Smartly, she followed up this observation by obtaining the temperature of a fresh urine sample.

Of course, today, the use of digital thermometers across the forehead would eliminate the possibility of factitious fever.

In the second case, diagnosis was quite straightforward. Anyone properly trained to examine a microscopic specimen of urine would recognize that the red cells were not of human origin.

CHAPTER 28

The Missing Teeth

There is no more difficult art to acquire than the art of observation, and for some men it is quite as difficult to record an observation in brief and plain language.

SIR WILLIAM OSLER

When I was an intern, a nurse called to inform me that a patient was having chills and to ask if I would come take a look at him. The patient had familial Mediterranean fever (FMF). When I saw the patient, I was intent on determining whether he was having true rigor (shaking chills) or just chilliness. I asked him whether his teeth chattered. He looked at me, developed a silly grin, and said, "Well, let's look in the drawer and find out." He opened the drawer of his bedside table and took out his false teeth!

I had failed to note that the patient had false teeth and was not wearing them at the time. I hadn't really looked at him. This was a good lesson learned. When the physician examines a patient, it should be with purpose and focus, not simply a casual glance.

Question:

1. *Can you recount some experiences where you looked but did not observe?*

Familial Mediterranean fever (FMF) is a rare hereditary inflammatory disorder most often affecting people from the eastern part of the Mediterranean Sea. Every few weeks or months, starting before adulthood, the patient with FMF becomes acutely ill with high fever and severe abdominal pain. Chest and joint pains may occur as well, since the disease affects all the membranes of the body. The patient is prostrate, unable to get out of bed, and begging for pain relief. Examination of the abdomen reveals findings typical of a ruptured abdominal organ, such as a perforated ulcer. If the diagnosis is not clear, surgeons will almost always advise immediate surgery. Just as dramatic as the onset of symptoms is their disappearance. In most cases, the symptoms suddenly disappear after forty-eight to seventy-two hours, and the patient returns to normal health, only to suffer the reappearance of the illness weeks or months later.

Obviously, this disease can be very debilitating. Imagine feeling well but living with the realization that every few weeks to months you will suddenly develop severe abdominal pain and be quite incapacitated for a number of days. In the 1970s, a colleague from my resident days found that colchicine, a drug used to treat gout, was quite effective in preventing or reducing attacks in FMF patients. What an influence this drug had on the lives of people with frequent attacks of this debilitating illness, allowing them to lead more normal lives.

The disease is due to a gene mutation. If only one gene is inherited, there are no symptoms. When two people with such a mutation have children, there is a 25 percent chance that any one child will receive the gene from both parents and thus have the disease. A genetic test is now available. Such a test is helpful in counseling couples who may be asymptomatic carriers of the mutant gene.

I admitted a patient with FMF one day. He was a man in his thirties, the diagnosis having been established a few years earlier. His findings were typical of FMF: severe abdominal and chest pain, temperature of 104 degrees, and a rigid, board-like abdomen with absent bowel sounds and rebound tenderness; a classic sign of a ruptured abdominal organ. Without asking me, my intern called for a surgical consult. The surgical chief resident came, examined the patient, and indicated that immediate exploratory surgery was called for. I said that the patient's findings were typical of his disease and that close observation was called for, not surgery. Neither my intern nor the surgical chief resident was comfortable with this watch-and-wait approach. Neither had ever managed a patient with FMF before.

I confirmed with the patient that his findings were typical of past acute episodes. He defused the conflict between me and the other residents by refusing to consider surgery. As expected, after about forty-eight hours the symptoms went away almost as rapidly as they had appeared, and the patient was discharged home.

Here is a classic example of the need to listen to the patient and involve him or her in medical decisions. Patients with chronic or recurring illness almost always know the fine points of their disease better than do the physicians caring for them.

Question:

1. *Have you had one or more patients who have chosen to disregard their doctor's advice for what they felt was a more appropriate path for them?*

CHAPTER 29

The Certifying Exam

All men by nature desire knowledge

ARISTOTLE

Certification as a specialist in internal medicine required satisfactory completion of a board examination (American Board of Internal Medicine), followed by an oral examination. There were two examiners for the orals, each of whom observed the board candidate take a medical history from a patient, examine the patient, reach a diagnosis, and suggest a treatment program.

My examination, in 1965, took place at the Boston VA hospital. My first examiner was a well- known physician from Philadelphia. I examined a patient who was in the hospital for evaluation of kidney failure. He had had his right kidney removed some years ago. He did not know the reason for the removal, and there were no records to clarify. When I presented the case to the examiner, I reviewed my bedside findings. He asked whether I could palpate the left kidney. I said I could not. He then examined the patient and indicated he could feel the left kidney. He suggested I follow his technique and try again. His technique was the same as mine. Again, I could not feel the kidney. I told him so and beneath my breath said, "Well, strike one."

We then went into a conference room where we reviewed his x-rays. The examiner placed an x-ray of the abdomen in the view box. I looked at the left kidney shadow and noted it could not be more than ten centimeters in length while saying to myself that a ten-centimeter kidney could not be felt at the bedside. I wasn't sure whether the examiner had been testing me or not when he said he could feel the left kidney, so I said nothing.

As he was removing the film, something caught my eye, and I asked him to put the film back in the view box. I looked, and lo and behold, there was the shadow of the right kidney just as plain as day. Obviously, it had not been removed. The examiner then went to the patient's record and reviewed the x-ray report. The radiologist had not picked up the fact that the patient's right kidney was still intact.

At that point the examiner put the patient's chart down, looked up, and asked, "Did you say you were from Philadelphia?" I replied yes. He then said, "What do you think of the Eagles' chances this season?" Instantly I knew that I had passed the examination. We spent the rest of the time gabbing about Philadelphia sports teams.

This story is one more example of becoming locked in with a thought pattern without questioning its accuracy. The radiologist had been informed that the patient had had his right kidney removed. He assumed this to be the case and neglected to examine the area where the right kidney would have been located.

The oral portion of the examination for certification in internal medicine was discontinued in the 1970s because of wide variation in the judgment of examiners. Today, such an examination would prove helpful in identifying deficiencies in "bedside" skills among today's young physicians—the ability to take a comprehensive history from a patient and perform a thorough physical examination.

Question:

1. *Have you observed something important about a patient that was missed by your resident or attending?*

CHAPTER 30

The Brioschi Man

The business of art is to reveal the relationship between man and his environment.

DAVID HERBERT LAWRENCE

During my residency years, one of my clinic patients was a pleasant, elderly Italian immigrant widower with chronic congestive heart failure. The patient showed up in the emergency room with great frequency, complaining of shortness of breath, weight gain, and swelling of his legs. These signs of congestive heart failure were always quickly reversed with intravenous diuretics and an extra dose of digitalis. Such findings suggested an excess of sodium in the diet, but the patient insisted that he was not only not using salt but that he was buying low sodium milk, bread, and other foods.

I asked if I might pay him a visit at his house. He readily agreed. So, one Saturday when I was off duty, I referred to my map of Boston and drove over to his house in Chelsea. He welcomed me and we shared some small talk over coffee in his kitchen. At some point, I glanced over at a kitchen counter and spied a box of Brioschi. I asked him whether he was using any of it. He said, "Yes, indeed. I use it all the time to relieve my indigestion."

Well, Brioschi is 44 percent sodium bicarbonate by weight! He was taking four to five tablespoons a day to relieve abdominal distress, thus ingesting an enormous amount of sodium. We discussed the relationship between his use of Brioschi and his frequent bouts of congestive heart failure. Maalox replaced his Brioschi and his indigestion was well controlled. More importantly, there were no further admissions to the emergency room with flagrant signs of heart failure.

One can learn a great deal by observing a patient in his or her own surroundings.

Question:

1. *Have you ever made a house call? Did you observe anything that could have been important for the patient's care that you wouldn't have been aware of if you hadn't visited the home?*

CHAPTER 31

Overlooking the Obvious

Every closed eye is not sleeping and every open eye is not seeing.

BILL COSBY

One afternoon, one of my residents asked if I would help him with one of his clinic patients. The resident was concerned that the young man had not been feeling well for some months and that he (the resident) might be missing something.

I walked into the examining room and the diagnosis was obvious. The patient's eyes were prominent and he had a pronounced stare. The whites of his eyes showed below his upper lid. He had a fine tremor of the hands. His thyroid gland was diffusely enlarged and could be observed when he swallowed. His pulse was rapid. Reflexes were hyperactive. The patient had hyperthyroidism, for certain. Thyroid function tests confirmed the diagnosis.

I followed the patient with the resident for the next two years. Treatment with thyroid-suppressing medication was effective, and he returned to normal health.

The resident was appalled that he had missed such an obvious diagnosis. He had been following the patient in the clinic for a full year prior to diagnosis. In retrospect, it was clear that the subtle changes in the patient's facial appearance, leading eventually to the classical signs of hyperthyroidism, had escaped the resident's detection. He needed only to step back, detach, and relook. When he did so, the diagnosis was obvious.

Question:

1. *Have you ever missed a diagnosis that, in retrospect, was obvious? What did you learn from the case?*

Exophthalmos is the Latin term that describes bulging eyes. Truly bulging eyeballs are seen most often in patients with long-standing hyperthyroidism. In some cases, the bulging eyes continue, even progress, despite successful treatment of the overactive thyroid gland. Extreme forms are referred to as malignant exophthalmos because of the resistant nature of the condition. I had such a patient once. One day, as he was walking through a doorway he hit the open door with his left shoulder. The left eye immediately popped out and came to rest on the upper portion of his cheek. Undaunted, he lifted the underside of his eyeball and it popped back into its socket. His vision was none the worse for wear.

CHAPTER 32

Life Anew

Faith and knowledge lean largely upon each other in the practice of medicine.

PETER MERE LATHAM

A woman in her early forties was referred to me by a family physician from an outlying community. She had come to his office with a lump in her neck. The lump was found to be an enlarged group of lymph nodes. A biopsy was performed on one of the nodes, and the pathology report indicated a malignant lymphoma. The patient was contacted and she and her husband returned to the family physician's office where he informed her of the diagnosis. When she asked what the treatment and prognosis would be, he told her that she would not likely have more than a few months to live. He arranged for her to see me for further evaluation and treatment. Upon meeting them, I was immediately impressed with their obvious care for each other.

This patient was referred at the beginning of the revolution in the treatment of patients with Hodgkin's disease and other lymphomas. Until then (mid-1960s), most of these patients died within five years. With a multiplicity of new chemotherapeutic drugs available and the introduction of new and improved irradiation techniques that could treat all the lymph node-bearing areas of the body, the outcome for these patients had improved dramatically. After examining the patient and reviewing the pathology slides, I indicated to the patient and her husband that while this particular form of lymphoma was not yet curable, she should be able to count on some years of active life and that the treatment would be quite well tolerated.

Preliminary arrangements were made for treatment and she and her husband left the office. As they were walking down the hall, I happened to step out of the office. Looking after them, I noted they were holding hands, and she was looking at him with a smile on her face that said, "We have some good time left after all." And they did.

One can learn a great deal by observing the patient as he or she walks into the office. Gait, demeanor, evidence of discomfort, and numerous other characteristics can be observed in this way. The physician may learn, as well, by observing patients as they leave, as this case illustrates. The classic text by Morgan and Engel, *The Clinical Approach to the Patient*, states it well: "The physician is constantly observant. From the time the doctor first meets the patient or walks into the room, he is studying him and his surroundings to learn clues to his disease, his personality, and the sources of his distress."[xxi]

Question:

1. *What important diagnostic clues have you picked up by simply observing a patient?*

CHAPTER 33

Listen, Look, Feel

Learn to see, learn to hear, learn to feel, learn to smell and know that by practice alone you become expert. Medicine is learned by the bedside and not in the classroom.

SIR WILLIAM OSLER

One year, as a visiting professor at a well-known academic medical center in the Southeast, I was escorted to teaching rounds by my host on the first day. Rounds began in the conference room. My normal habit was to start rounds at the bedside of the patient, but I didn't say anything at the time. The intern presented the patient's medical history, then the physical examination, and before I knew it, he was reciting the findings of diagnostic tests and procedures. I halted him and suggested that we see the patient before hearing more.

At the bedside, I was introduced to a pleasant, matronly black woman. After spending a few minutes to confirm her medical history and check her heart and lungs, I focused on her abdominal examination. Standing at the end of the bed, the sheet folded down to the patient's lower abdomen, I observed a mass appearing in the left upper abdomen each time she inspired. The mass disappeared on each exhalation. Obviously, as the diaphragm moved downward with inspiration, it was pushing a mass toward the surface of the abdomen. Almost certainly, this was an enlarged spleen.

In theory, it could have been a large liver located on the "wrong" side, situs inversus, a congenital anomaly characterized by a reversal of the location of the body's internal organs. I knew that this was not the case, having examined the heart and noted its location on the left side. To be seen on inspection of the abdomen, the spleen would have to be between ten to twenty times normal size. Few conditions could result in a spleen of this size. I then went to the side of the bed and palpated the left side of the abdomen. The firm edge of this huge mass was easily felt and a splenic notch identified, an inverted V where the blood vessels leading to the spleen are located.

The intern had neither observed nor felt this mass. After I had him and the other members of the resident group examine the mass, I asked them what they thought it could be. Their responses were disappointing. Some suggested retroperitoneal tumors or other masses, such as a polycystic kidney, none of which would be expected to move with respiration. None were comfortable concluding that this was a massively enlarged spleen without obtaining a scan to confirm its presence and to rule out other causes of a left upper quadrant abdominal mass. The scan, of course, confirmed the presence of this huge spleen.

Questions:

1. *What other lesions should be included in the differential diagnosis of this mass?*
2. *What physical findings indicated that the mass was the spleen?*

Learners need to be reassured about their clinical decisions. It was disappointing to me, however, that the need for medical students and residents to recognize the value of good bedside observations was so undervalued by the faculty of this medical center. Would these learners always be in a clinical setting where the latest in medical imaging would be instantly available? And how often might they be able to avoid specialized tests and procedures by being more confident in their bedside skills?

Today's graduating medical students are so deficient in these skills that special courses have been developed for interns and residents at teaching hospitals across the country to learn what they should have learned in medical school. Even so, one rarely sees a young physician today who can comfortably arrive at a diagnosis without a battery of tests.

During this same visit, the next morning we had "walk" rounds, briefly visiting each patient on the floor. In one room, I observed a written note behind the head of the bed that read, "Fluid restriction—1,500 cc." The patient was convalescing from a mild heart attack and appeared to be doing well. I asked the resident team why the patient was on fluid restriction. They responded that all patients who come in with heart attacks are placed on salt and fluid restriction.

We learn in physiology that the kidneys do a fine job of salt (sodium) and water balance. When the salt concentration gets too low, the kidney excretes an excess of water. When the concentration is high, water is retained. Occasionally, in patients with heart failure and a few other conditions, the brain secretes an excess of an antidiuretic hormone. In such cases, excess water is retained and the sodium content of plasma is diluted. In extreme cases, convulsions may ensue. So, water restriction is indeed indicated in these patients. The only other condition that would mimic this situation is psychogenic water-drinking, a serious disorder characterized by the compulsion to drink water far in excess of the body's need.

The patient under discussion had normal kidney function and his electrolyte pattern indicated a normal sodium level. Hence, there was no reason to restrict fluids. I asked him how he was feeling, and he indicated that all was well—except that he was thirsty! Of course he was thirsty. Restricting water in a patient with normal fluid balance would be expected to result, ultimately, in thirst.

This is an example of a pattern of care at this medical center for patients with heart attacks that became established dogma without any physiologic basis. There are many other patterns of care at various teaching hospitals that have no rational explanation, patterns that have been carried down through generations of physicians in training whose teachers have not been sufficiently observant to correct them.

Question:

1. *Can you identify a "standardized" pattern of care at your hospital or clinic that has no basis in fact?*

CHAPTER 34

The Silent Tumor

He is the best physician who is the most ingenious inspirer of hope.

SAMUEL TAYLOR COLERIDGE

One Saturday morning, an intern asked if I would see his wife. He was concerned about the appearance of mild but diffuse swelling of her neck and face. He had asked his teaching attending physician to see her. The attending had assured him that there was nothing to worry about, that her thyroid was normal. The intern's wife had no symptoms and was not aware of swelling of the neck or face. On my examination, her neck veins were bulging, and when I raised her hands above the level of the heart, the veins did not empty.

These findings were characteristic of obstruction of the superior vena cava, the huge vein that accepts drainage of the venous blood from the entire body and empties into the right side of the heart. The blood is then transported to the lung to pick up oxygen, returned to the left side of the heart, and sent out to the rest of the body for its cells to accept the vital oxygen. In a young patient in good health, by far the most common cause is a tumor in the central portion of the chest compressing the thin wall of the vena cava and holding up the drainage of blood from the body's veins. We arranged for the patient to obtain a chest x-ray. It showed a huge tumor occupying the center of her thorax.

A biopsy of this tumor confirmed the suspicion that she had Hodgkin's disease. A series of studies suggested that there was no evidence that the tumor involved other lymphatic organs of the body. Ordinarily, her treatment (at the time) would have involved irradiation to all the lymph node-bearing areas of the body, first the nodes above the diaphragm followed by those below. However, the patient was four months pregnant. Irradiation below the diaphragm would have resulted in the death of the fetus.

The radiation oncologists urged the patient to have an abortion. The patient was very reluctant to pursue this path. She wanted this child. She, her husband, and I had a series of conversations about possible alternatives. I indicated that I thought it was possible that deferring irradiation below the diaphragm until after the child was born could still result in a cure. Certainly, this approach would increase the risk of a recurrence of her disease. There were no published data to guide us on this issue. Despite intense disagreement by the staff of the radiation oncology department, we chose this path. She received irradiation to all the lymph node-bearing areas above the diaphragm, and then awaited the birth of her child. A healthy boy came into the world after a normal birth process. Eight weeks later, irradiation of the lymph node-bearing areas below the diaphragm was begun. Her ovaries were protected as well as possible in the event that the patient and her husband wished to have another child.

The story has a good ending. It is now thirty-two years later. The patient remains well and the child, born between cycles of irradiation, is a healthy adult. And—oh, yes—the couple had two more children.

Here is an example of the tendency of many specialists to fail to see the whole patient. The specialist who saw the patient initially narrowed his attention to the thyroid, missing the obvious distention of her neck veins, a sure sign of a deeper problem.

Questions:

2. *Have you been in a situation where there was a strong difference of opinion between physicians about the best course of treatment?*
3. *What would you do if you knew that an inappropriate treatment was planned?*

CHAPTER 35

The Murmur That Was

It is what we know already that prevents us from learning.

CLAUDE BERNARD

During my second year of medical school, when we first were introduced to the stethoscope, I placed my scope on the chest of a classmate, Ted. I detected a murmur and asked the instructor to listen. He did and pronounced it a benign flow murmur. Neither of us thought any more of it.

Some years later, my family and I drove to Oberlin, Ohio, to spend the Thanksgiving holiday with Ted and his family. In the course of the visit, he asked if I would do a physical on him. He said he was having severe headaches. He had had a checkup recently but was not satisfied with the appointment.

We went over to the clinic. I asked about the nature of the headaches then examined him. The blood pressure in his right arm was 250/140!

In the left, it was 100/50. The pressures were only slightly higher in the legs than in the left arm. Examination of his eyes with an ophthalmoscope showed changes due to hypertension. A loud systolic murmur was heard at the base of the heart, the same murmur that was heard twelve years earlier. No further examination was necessary. These findings could have only one explanation; a blockage of the aorta after the right brachial and carotid arteries but before the left brachial. Such a blockage is almost always due to a congenital narrowing of the aorta, referred to as a coarctation.

An x-ray of the chest showed the classical findings of rib notching due to enlargement of the intercostal arteries, nature's attempt to find a detour around the blockage. Arrangements were made for Ted to undergo surgery at a well-known hospital to have the coarctation repaired. The aorta was clamped, the area of narrowing removed, and a Teflon graft inserted to bridge the gap. His blood pressures returned to normal, and the headaches disappeared. Unfortunately, his larynx was injured during the procedure and his voice did not return for about a year. He resumed his practice, however, and lived well into his seventh decade.

The diagnosis of coarctation of the aorta is usually made prior to adulthood. That Ted was able to remain healthy in the face of this defect until almost forty years of age is quite unusual.

Here is an example of a serious diagnosis overlooked at least twice (with potentially lethal consequences) by the failure to perform a proper examination. The diagnosis of an innocuous murmur after a superficial examination by the medical school instructor might be excused. Certainly not to be excused, however, was the failure to identify the problem at the time of his checkup prior to our visit. The blood pressure would have been abnormal regardless of which arm was used, signaling the need to check the pressure in the other arm. The diagnosis would then have been obvious.

Questions:

1. *What are the characteristics of an innocent murmur as opposed to a clinically significant murmur?*
2. *Can one be confident in distinguishing one from another without further study?*
3. *What procedure would you order to distinguish between an innocent and a clinically significant murmur?*

CHAPTER 36

Nails

For days after death, hair and fingernails continue to grow but phone calls taper off.

JOHNNY CARSON

When I was an intern, I admitted an elderly patient with vague symptoms of fatigue and weakness. On physical examination, her fingernails had white discolorations. I paid no more attention to them until my resident and I were at a loss to explain the patient's symptoms. I found myself looking at her nails again and asked how long they had looked like that. She replied that they had been that way for two to three years.

I went to the library to learn more about diseased nails and found a picture of fingernails that were identical to those of my patient. They were Plummer's nails, described many years ago in patients with hyperthyroidism by a physician whose name became attached to the abnormality. My patient had no overt symptoms or signs of hyperthyroidism, but a check of her thyroid hormone levels showed they were quite high. She had what is known as apathetic hyperthyroidism, a very subtle form of the disease noted most often in elderly patients. She was treated with radioactive iodine and responded quite nicely. She moved away after about three months, and I never knew whether her nails returned to normal.

Nails grow slowly. It takes about four months for the portion of the nail that starts at the base to arrive at the end of the finger. Nail abnormalities are often a clue to unrecognized underlying disease.[xxii] Fingernails that are concave, known as spooned nails (koilonychia), may be seen in patients with long-standing iron deficiency. A more common finding in iron-deficient patients is paleness of the nails. Nails that are excessively broad, rounded, and lifted off their base (clubbing) may be a clue to unrecognized cancer of the lung. Other forms of lung or heart disease may also cause this finding.

Nails that show thin, red, vertical, parallel lines (splinter hemorrhages) are seen in patients with vascular diseases such as lupus erythematosus. In patients with unexplained fever, this nail finding may be a clue to smoldering bacterial endocarditis. The lunula (half moon) of the nail may disappear in patients with liver disease. Evenly spaced transverse depressions in the nail (Mees' or Beau's lines), occurring at the same spot on all the nails, may be caused by any serious illness that results in inhibition of growth. Nails normally grow about 3 mm per month. Measuring the distance from the nail bed to the depression provides an estimate of the illness that caused them. Today, chemotherapy is the most frequent cause of Mees' lines. Arsenic poisoning may cause them, a clue sometimes referred to in who-done-it novels of yesteryear.

Pairs of symmetrical, horizontal white lines parallel to the lunula are known as Muehrcke's lines. They disappear on compression of the nail. They occur at times when blood protein (albumin) levels are low, as seen in some patients with renal or liver disease or malnutrition.

Dark longitudinal streaks in the nails are seen in most blacks. In older persons of color, newly developing pigmented lines in a single nail should arouse suspicion of melanoma.

Blue (azure) lunulae are seen in patients with Wilson's disease, a congenital abnormality of copper metabolism. A similar colored ring around the iris of the eye (Kayser-Fleischer ring) is seen in this condition. Finally, the nails may take on a ground glass appearance in some patients with severe liver disease.

I cite these examples of systemic diseases that may be suspected from close examination of the fingernails to point to the great value of close observation when examining a patient.

Question:

1. *What other systemic diagnoses can be suspected by closely examining the entire hand?*

PART THREE

Learning Moments from Other Stories

It wasn't until the 1960s that medical technologies became available to treat a number of chronic illnesses which, in time, would otherwise prove fatal. Examples include valve replacement therapy for rheumatic heart disease, dialysis and kidney transplantation for chronic renal failure, and transfusion of blood products such as platelets and white blood cells for bleeding problems and infections. With a wealth of diagnostic and therapeutic technologies readily available, today's physicians rarely have the opportunity to observe the body's remarkable ability to adapt to serious chronic disease, too often resulting in overtreatment or treating when it is not necessary. "Tincture of time" is one therapy that is underused. The first four stories in this section (chapters 37 through 40) of the book are examples of how effectively the body can adapt to otherwise life-threatening chronic illness.

Patients with incurable diseases live with the realization that they will soon leave their loved ones behind. The next three chapters (41 through 43) stuck with me over the years as being particularly good examples of how much we can learn from patients as they prepare for death. Their poise, courage, and concern for their families have always been an inspiration for me. Medical and nursing students can experience this only by being able to follow such patients over extended periods.

Chapters 44 through 47 help one understand that humorous episodes with patients help make medicine such a rewarding profession. These episodes help physicians put their own world into perspective by observing how patients maintain their sense of humor under the most adverse circumstances.

At the end of his or her career, every physician can recall stories of the kind I've shared in this book—stories that represent learning moments, stories that reinforce the importance of basic skills, stories that bring a smile or a laugh. But always, one or two stories stand alone in the physician's memory bank for their significance. The last story in this part of the book (chapter 48) is the one I remember most vividly.

CHAPTER 37

Rusty Blood

The art of medicine consists in amusing the patient while nature cures the disease.

VOLTAIRE

One day during my internship, I was called to the emergency room to admit a patient with severe anemia. The patient was a thirty-nine-year-old woman who, twenty years earlier, had become convinced that iron was bad for her. So, after studying the iron content of various foods, she had carefully avoided anything known to contain iron.

Iron, of course, is necessary to produce hemoglobin, the protein that permits red blood cells to carry oxygen to the tissues of the body. Indeed, all body cells require iron, not only red cells. Iron absorbed in excess of cellular requirements is stored in the liver. Body stores of iron average about two grams. But, during childbearing years, women lose up to 2 percent of their iron stores each month, the result of blood loss during their menstrual periods. A balanced diet provides a sufficient amount of iron to keep pace with these monthly losses. A quick calculation will show, however, that for most women, the lack of dietary iron would result in iron deficiency within a few short years. Since it is not possible to totally exclude iron from the diet, deficiency could take longer, but certainly not twenty years. Thus, this patient was almost certainly severely deficient.

Anemia is the most evident result of iron deficiency and this was indeed the case. The patient was so pale that anemia was almost certainly profound. Blood counts confirmed this. Her hemoglobin level was 1.5 g/dL! She had less than 15 percent of the normal amount of hemoglobin, the oxygen-carrying protein in red cells. Indeed, when I drew a blood sample from her to determine her blood counts, the blood sample looked like rusty water instead of the thick, dark red-appearing normal blood. Her red blood cell count was 600,000/uL. Normal for a woman would be about four million. Here was a patient with almost 90 percent of her oxygen-carrying capacity lacking who had actually walked into the emergency room!

When iron deficiency anemia is present, oxygen is carried and delivered more efficiently to the body's cells than in patients who are not anemic. This is the result of an increase in both the rate of breathing and the heartbeat. So, more oxygen is carried by the red blood cells to the tissues of the body. In addition, the percent of oxygen released by these cells at the tissue level is increased. My patient's heart rate was about 120/minute, and her respirations were 30/minute, about twice normal. Her lungs were "wet" with fluid and she had striking swelling of the legs. It was clear that her body had accommodated about as far as it could and was now failing her.

Incredibly, we did not transfuse this patient. At the time, in 1960, Boston was suffering from an unacceptably high rate of hepatitis among blood donors. One of every six or seven patients receiving blood was developing hepatitis. And, of course, tests for antibodies to hepatitis had not yet been developed. So, after consulting with the patient, we elected not to transfuse her and relied on daily doses of oral iron to correct her anemia. And, wow, was her body ready to use the iron! At the end of the first week of treatment, her bone marrow was turning out red blood cells at sixty times the normal rate.

The patient remained in the hospital for about three weeks. She received counseling about the importance of iron, the signs of heart failure disappeared, and her anemia was mostly corrected by the time she was discharged. She was a totally different woman from the one who had entered the hospital, near death, three weeks earlier.

This is a fine example of the ability of the human body, given time, to adapt to extreme circumstances. It reinforces the importance of moderation in the treatment of patients whose bodies have adjusted to long-standing medical problems. In these instances, the tendency is great to correct the problem immediately. A slow but steady treatment plan is the order of the day.

Question:

1. *What are some other illnesses that should be reversed slowly?*

CHAPTER 38

Plugging Holes

Time is generally the best doctor.

OVID

Thrombocytopenic purpura is the term used to describe bleeding from a deficiency of platelets, microscopic bodies that serve to plug tiny holes in capillaries. There are many known causes of thrombocytopenia, such as leukemia, bone marrow failure, immunologic disorders, adverse drug reactions, and marked enlargement of the spleen. Idiopathic thrombocytopenic purpura (ITP) is the term used when there is no obvious cause of the low platelets. Most often, an immune mechanism is at play, since such patients usually respond to treatment with corticosteroids and other immunosuppressive drugs.

Platelets normally live in the circulation for seven to eight days. Young platelets are more effective as clotting agents than older ones. In ITP, platelets are destroyed by antibodies relatively soon after they enter the circulation, sometimes in a matter of hours. A normal platelet count is between 150,000–250,000/uL. In ITP, the count may fall as low as 10,000/uL, sometimes even lower. At these levels, patients are at great risk of life-threatening bleeding, such as cerebral or gastrointestinal hemorrhage. Platelet transfusions are generally not helpful, since transfused platelets become damaged from the patient's antibodies in much the same fashion as with her own platelets.

Most cases of ITP are fairly short-lived. They either disappear spontaneously or are cured with corticosteroids or removal of the spleen. In some instances, ITP persists as a chronic condition. I was referred such a patient in the late 1960s, a young girl fourteen years of age. Susan had been treated at another hospital and had not responded to either corticosteroids or splenectomy. Her platelet count fluctuated between 10,000–15,000/uL. Despite the very low count, the amount of bleeding she noted was remarkably mild. A few bruises and petechiae (tiny hemorrhages into the skin, no larger than a pinhead) were all that could be observed. We labeled her blood platelets with a radioactive agent (chromium 51) and re-injected them to determine how long they survived. Her platelets survived in her circulation for less than two hours, becoming sequestered in the liver, ordinarily a very inefficient organ for removing damaged platelets from the blood.

I followed Susan for twenty-seven years, first weekly, then monthly, then quarterly, and then twice a year. Remarkably, she never required hospitalization, despite the fact that her platelet count never exceeded 20,000/uL. She never had a heavy menstrual flow, nosebleed, or bleeding from other common sites. I shouldn't have been surprised. After all, her platelets were only a few hours old. They were most efficient in plugging holes.

Susan became a nurse. She never married. We would have been challenged had she married and become pregnant. Not only would we have been concerned about hemorrhage before or during childbirth, we would have anticipated that the infant would be born with thrombocytopenia.

Antibodies, you see, cross the placenta. In such instances, if the infant survives the first few weeks of life, a normal platelet count can be anticipated once the maternal antibody is cleared from the child's blood.

Here again, is an example of the body's extraordinary ability to adapt to serious, nonmalignant disorders that evolve over many years.

Questions:

1. *What are the most serious bleeding complications resulting from a low platelet count?*
2. *What hereditary bleeding disorder is made worse with the use of aspirin? Why?*

CHAPTER 39

Forty-Eight Pounds in Forty-Eight Hours

In youth, the days are short and years are long. In old age, the years are short and days long.

POPE PAUL VI

During my internship, an elderly woman was admitted to my ward with the diagnosis of congestive heart failure. After taking her medical history and performing a physical examination, I was astounded that the woman was still alive. She had an enormous amount of edema, from her feet all the way up to her breasts. She had to sit upright in order to breathe. She had large pleural effusions—fluid on the outside of both lungs. Her heart sounds were distant and muffled.

It was not clear what the cause of her heart failure was, but it *was* clear that her very survival depended upon relieving her of the massive accumulation of fluid. I had the nurse administer 2 cc of Mercuhydrin, a potent diuretic agent. Within the hour, the patient began to void large amounts of urine. Indeed, over the next forty-eight hours, she lost forty-eight pounds, all water. She was on the bedpan constantly and begged us to stop doing what we were doing to make her pee. Of course, having given her the Mercuhydrin, we could not reverse its effect.

Finally, she had relief from the constant urination. By this time, her edema had disappeared, the pleural effusions had vanished, and we could now hear crisp heart sounds. Indeed, we heard an additional heart sound, an opening snap, the classical finding in patients with mitral stenosis. For many years, her damaged mitral valve must have been slowly reducing her cardiac output and causing blood to back up. Finally, her body could not compensate and heart failure developed. Heart failure is the term used to describe the accumulation of fluid (plasma) that leaks out of capillaries in the lungs and lower extremities because of the pressure within these capillaries from the increased amount of blood that has backed up.

When we obtained an x-ray during this woman's convalescence, we determined why she had compensated for so many years. She had a giant left atrium. It was so large it took up three-fourths of the space in her chest. The atrium had slowly enlarged to accommodate the blood that was not getting into the left ventricle because of the stenotic mitral valve. This giant atrium had thus protected the lungs and the venous system from the complications of blood backing up. Only after many, many years did the atrium itself fail, the result being the slowly increasing amount of edema that finally accumulated to an extreme extent. Further history revealed that during adolescence, the patient had had a prolonged episode of fever with swollen joints throughout her body—classic signs of rheumatic fever and the cause of the damaged mitral valve.

Surgical correction of rheumatic valvular disease was in its infancy when this patient was hospitalized. She was considered too high a surgical risk to undergo the valvulotomy procedure available at the time. She returned home and lived a moderately restricted but enjoyable life before dying two years later from refractory heart failure.

Questions:

1. *Why do we no longer see many cases of rheumatic heart disease in this country?*
2. *How would you have treated this patient to avoid the massive, abrupt loss of fluid?*

Today's physicians rarely see patients with such advanced illnesses. Annual medical examinations and routine blood tests all contribute to earlier detection of chronic conditions. Thank goodness for that. A downside of earlier diagnosis, however, is that young physicians often fail to appreciate the extraordinary ability of the body to adapt to serious physical, biochemical, or hormonal problems when they evolve over a long period. The result is a tendency to rush in and correct the problem overnight. This case is one such example. If we had simply placed the patient at bed rest and salt restriction only, she would have lost much of that fluid in a less stressful way.

CHAPTER 40

A Life Taken

A mother's love is patient and forgiving when all others are forsaking, it never fails or falters, even though the heart is breaking.

Helen Rice

One of my patients, George, was a nineteen year old young man with acute leukemia. George was a hell-raiser. He left high school without graduating. He did not seek a job. He drank, smoked, and ran with a bad crowd. His mother was a single parent. She was frustrated and sad that he had turned out so poorly.

In the 1960s, acute myelogenous leukemia was not curable. Most patients died within six months of diagnosis. Quality of life during the course of their illness was not good. Infections, bleeding, bad side effects of chemotherapy, and repeated hospitalizations were the rule.

George and I developed a healthy rapport. He took his medications on schedule. He called promptly when he was in need. He distanced himself from his unsavory friends. Eventually, after one of many prolonged hospitalizations, I indicated that we had little more to offer except to help him be comfortable. He said he would like to go home to die.

After returning home, he survived for quite some weeks, much longer than I had expected. I visited him each evening on my way home from the hospital. We chatted and I felt he was accepting his fate with courage and dignity. Then I received the call from his mother that he had died.

After the funeral, which I attended, she asked if I would come by the house one more time. I did and she presented me with an unfinished painting of snow-covered mountains. It was quite a good painting. George had painted it and was going to present it to me, but he had died before completing it. I was dumbstruck. Here was a young man who had changed from an incorrigible adolescent to a sensitive, caring person in the space of just a few months. His mother's grief over his passing was muted by this wonderful transformation.

Moments such as these are what make the profession of medicine so rewarding. Disappointment over the inability to extend this boy's life was balanced, in part, by the realization that his terminal illness brought him back to his mother.

Question:

3. *Have you ever received a gift from a patient? How did you respond to the patient? What did you do with the gift?*

CHAPTER 41

Misinterpreting an Important Test

The only real mistake is the one from which we learn nothing.

JOHN POWELL

The spring of 1962 brought a twenty-five-year-old airman across the country to be evaluated for a disability incurred while he was on active duty. He traveled by train. He vomited repeatedly during the trip. By the time he reached Washington, DC, he was so weak he had to be transported from the train to the Andrews Air Force Base hospital by ambulance. I was called to see him in the emergency room.

One of my residents was with me when we arrived. The airman was almost unresponsive. His eyes were turned toward the ceiling. He was too weak to move. He had a pulse of forty-two and a blood pressure of 64/0. It was clear that he had only minutes to live. I had the resident insert an IV consisting of normal saline to which an ampule of glucose was added. In addition, he was given a shot of cortisone. Both glucose and cortisone can be life-saving in situations such as this and will not hurt when not needed.

While the resident was doing this, I quickly pored over the thick medical record the patient had brought with him. He had been tested a few weeks earlier in Denver, Colorado, for weakness, low blood glucose, and persistent nausea. Among the diagnostic possibilities was Addison's disease, insufficiency of the adrenal gland. The twenty-four-hour urine specimen he submitted to the laboratory to evaluate adrenal function showed borderline levels of hydroxyl- steroids, compounds produced by the adrenal. He was then correctly given ACTH, a pituitary hormone that stimulates adrenal production. A repeat twenty-four-hour urine sample was then tested for the same metabolites. The results were identical: borderline normal. It was falsely concluded that his adrenal gland was functioning satisfactorily, a critical mistake. The repeat study of the adrenal compounds should have shown a doubling or tripling of the baseline levels after ACTH stimulation!

It was then obvious to us that the patient did indeed have Addison's disease and that the trip across the country with nausea, vomiting, and inadequate fluid replacement had precipitated an "Addisonian crisis." Such a crisis can be reversed remarkably quickly. There are few diseases in humans that can cause a patient to swing from near death one moment to perfectly normal the next. Acute Addison's disease is one. Indeed, by the time I had completed my review of the record, the patient's blood pressure and pulse had returned to normal, he was feeling stronger, and was sitting up. Within an hour, he was up and about, almost as though nothing had happened.

We kept him in the hospital for a few days to repeat the studies he had had in Denver. They confirmed the diagnosis, and, with a modest daily replacement dose of cortisone, the patient returned to a normal life. Since the illness occurred while he was on active duty, he received a discharge from the air force with a partial disability pension.

We contacted the physician in Denver who had misinterpreted the findings from the urinary studies and brought him up to date, as diplomatically as possible, about the patient's course of events. He responded angrily and dismissed the life-threatening event as grandstanding. I was disappointed that he did not view this as a learning opportunity.

In medicine, the old adage "If it ain't broke, don't fix it" has been replaced by "If it isn't perfect, let's keep working toward that." Only through such a philosophy can the quality of patient care be continuously improved.

Question:

1. *In a patient brought into an emergency room who appears to be near death, what is the single most important immediate step to take that may be lifesaving?*

CHAPTER 42

About Courage

The doctor knows what his trained eyes see and he says it's the last of the ninth for me. So one more thing while the clouds loom dark and then I must leave this noisy park.

ANONYMOUS

One of my first patients, Mrs. S, was a pleasant forty-five-year old woman who had chronic myelogenous leukemia (CML). She was the wife of a senior noncommissioned officer. She had had the disease for about three years and was requiring very little treatment.

CML is an illness that tends to evolve in stages. In many patients, the first few years after the diagnosis is established are often quiescent—the "good" phase. During this period, white blood cells slowly accumulate in the bone marrow and are reflected by increasing cell counts in the blood. Other blood counts tend to remain stable. The patient has no symptoms and is able to function normally. Without treatment, the white cell count may increase to as much as twenty to forty times normal. At these levels, there is a risk that the cells will clog up small capillaries, leading to the loss of blood supply to vital organs. Fortunately, one or more chemotherapeutic drugs called alkylating agents, taken by mouth, are remarkably effective in reducing the white cell count to normal, with few or no side effects. Mrs. S was taking a small dose of such a drug, Busulfan.

When I next saw her, she complained of difficulty urinating. Examination of the lower abdomen revealed a distended urinary bladder. On pelvic examination, a rock-hard mass was felt at the level of the cervix. Such a mass, in this location, usually indicates advanced cancer of the cervix. I was distressed for Mrs. S. First CML and now advanced cervical cancer. I arranged for an ob-gyn colleague to obtain a biopsy of the mass. Imagine my surprise (and relief) when the biopsy report showed the mass to be an accumulation of white blood cells! Massive numbers of these cells had escaped from the blood and formed a gradually enlarging mass at the base of the bladder and the uterus. A "tumor" made up of nothing but white cells is an extremely rare complication of CML. It is referred to as a chloroma. Fortunately, such tumors are very sensitive to x-ray therapy. I arranged for Mrs. S to receive radiation treatments, and the tumor melted away promptly, as did her urinary symptoms.

She was quite stable for another year. Then, the accelerated phase of her leukemia began. In the 1960s, the onset of this phase in patients with CML predicted death within six to nine months. The bone marrow either converted to a form of acute leukemia or stopped producing blood cells normally. In Mrs. S's case, her blood counts began to fall.

Today's technology allows for white blood cells, red cells, platelets, and plasma components to be separated individually and made available to patients. Further, the development of bone marrow transplantation now makes it possible to transplant such patients before the disease reaches the accelerated phase. So, in the 1960s, while the anemia that developed could be controlled with red blood cell transfusions, the lack of blood platelets (the tiny cells that plug microscopic holes in capillaries) could not be corrected. Mrs. S's platelet count slowly fell to dangerously low levels.

By the Christmas season of 1962, she began to show bleeding into the skin and had had a number of nosebleeds. On Christmas Eve morning, she awoke with a headache. She asked her husband not to leave for his work at Andrews Air Force Base. When the children were up and had

had breakfast, she told them she was feeling poorly and suggested they celebrate Christmas a day early. The family enjoyed the morning opening their presents and sipping hot chocolate. Around noon, Mrs. S decided to lie down for a rest. Within the hour, she had slipped into a coma. Her husband arranged for her to be transported to the hospital, where an examination showed that she had suffered a massive cerebral hemorrhage. She died quietly later that day.

I have never forgotten the quiet dignity of Mrs. S nor her prescience in bringing the family together to celebrate Christmas early. She was a courageous woman. It is important for physicians to reflect on their experiences with such patients. Recalling such stories tends to balance physicians' frustration and anger over being unable to cure patients or prevent their deaths.

Exercise:

1. *Write about a patient incident you've witnessed that has reinforced your commitment to "cure sometimes, to help always."*

CHAPTER 43

Faith

Drugs are not always necessary. Belief in recovery always is.

NORMAN COUSINS

In the early 1970s, I was referred an elderly woman from an outlying community. She was a retired schoolteacher, a lovely lady. She had chronic lymphatic leukemia. Most patients with this disease live for quite some years, eight to nine years after diagnosis, on average. During this time, relatively little treatment is generally needed, just simple oral chemotherapy with minimal side effects. Often, as in the case with this patient, no treatment is needed during the early years of the disease. Her red cell and platelet counts were normal. Her only risk was of infection, given that the number of normal white blood cells was lower than normal.

For the first couple of years, I had her return every six months. Thereafter, because her blood counts were so stable, I saw her just once a year. Our visits were always pleasant. While not particularly religious, the patient had faith. She carried a positive outlook, enjoying travel and bridge with her friends and reading.

One visit, about in her eleventh year after diagnosis, the blood counts were back to normal. I repeated the blood work to be sure, and—yes, indeed—all traces of the chronic leukemia had disappeared. A bone marrow examination confirmed the disappearance of the leukemia. I remember being so pleased to be able to share with this lovely lady that her illness had resolved by itself. She welcomed this news.

I kept track of her for some years through her local physician. She remained healthy for quite a long time, ultimately dying of "old age" without any sign of leukemia ever recurring.

There are many, many stories of patients whose otherwise fatal illnesses disappeared spontaneously. Either immunologic or psychologic factors (or both) may be responsible for spontaneous regression of cancer. In many cases, disappearance of the cancer follows an acute febrile episode. Faith may have much to do with these remarkable stories. We have much to learn about the factors responsible for spontaneous remission.

In his book *Love, Medicine, and Miracles: Lessons Learned About Self-Healing from a Surgeon's Experience with Exceptional Patients*, Dr. Bernie Siegel describes how patients with cancer who are able to laugh and play, and who enjoy living, live longer and have greater life satisfaction than those who do not.[xxiii] His writings reinforce the importance of mind/body relationships in the outcomes of patients with serious illnesses. These writings validate the pioneering work of Dr. Robert Ader, who showed that emotions have a powerful impact on the body's immune system.[xxiv] Enhancement of the body's immune response to disease is thought by many to explain why patients with a positive outlook on life tend to be more functional and live longer.

Question:

1. *Have you had a patient, family member, or friend whose fatal illness just went away? How was the spontaneous recovery explained?*

CHAPTER 44

Delicate Moments

A sense of humor is the ability to understand a joke and that the joke is on oneself.

CLIFTON FADIMAN

One morning during my second year of residency, a well-dressed elderly woman entered the emergency room with the complaint of abdominal pain. She lived on Beacon Hill, just a few minutes away. Her internist was not available that day. It was a Thursday. In the 1950s and '60s, it was fashionable for personal physicians to take Thursdays off.

I took the lady's medical history. It was quite unremarkable. Equally so was her abdominal examination. Still not clear what her problem was, I indicated that I would like to perform an internal examination. She said OK. With the assistance of a nurse, I performed the pelvic examination. Midway through the examination, she turned her head toward me and in a pleasant, gentle voice asked, "Young man, does your mother know what you do for a living?"

A few years later, my first year in practice, I was performing a pelvic examination on a middle-aged woman in the early evening. The examination room did not have a window. Neither did I have an attendant present. In the middle of the examination, the lights suddenly went off. The woman sat bolt upright on the examination table and asked, "OK, buster, what's next?" Frantic, I rushed out to get the nurse only to find that the entire office was dark.

The great blackout of the Northeast had just occurred (October, 1965). All of New York State and much of New Jersey, Rhode Island, and Connecticut had been affected from the outage, which had started at a power plant at Niagara Falls, New York. Of course, we didn't know that at the time, but the patient was reassured that I was not the cause of the sudden darkness.

I learned an important lesson from that experience, to always have an aide present when performing a pelvic examination—for the reassurance of both the patient and physician.

Question:

1. *How helpful is the pelvic examination as a screening procedure in asymptomatic women?*

CHAPTER 45

The Local Pharmacist

Always laugh when you can. It is cheap medicine.

LORD BYRON

One of my patients was an elderly woman from Corning, New York, who had a chronic refractory anemia. Periodically, she had to be admitted to receive two to three units of blood. Over the years of her illness, she came to know the staff of the hospital quite well. Of course, she came into contact with many interns and residents. This woman had an amazing plethora of jokes, many quite racy. Only after getting to know a new intern or resident fairly well would she risk sharing a racy joke or two with him or her.

One morning, an intern and I were visiting her. Toward the end of our visit, she turned to the intern and said that she felt he was mature enough to hear one of her stories. She said, "A few days before coming into the hospital, I had to go to my druggist, George. I said, 'George, I need some hair remover.' So he rummaged around and pulled a bottle off the shelf. He gave me the bottle and said if it was for under my arms, I should dilute a portion of the contents with water, half and half, and apply it twice a day. But if it was for my face, I should dilute it one in four and put it on only once a day. I said, 'No, George, the hair remover is for my schnauzer.' He then said, 'Oh, in that case, use it undiluted, three times a day, and don't ride your bike for a week.'"

I have always been amazed at the ability of patients to retain their sense of humor in the face of serious illness. This woman of almost ninety years was a wonderful example of how humor transcends discomfort and a bleak future.

Exercise:

1. *Record some humorous events that you've witnessed during your clinical rotations. Have any of them helped defuse a tough situation?*

CHAPTER 46

The Brigadier General

If you lose the power to laugh, you lose the power to think.

CLARENCE DARROW

Herm Ortle, an endocrinologist, was one of my air force physician colleagues. He had little regard for the spit and polish of the military. He was a fine physician with a great sense of humor. One day, while walking across the base, he was pulled up short by a major general who said, "You're out of uniform, Captain." Herm asked, "What do you mean?" The general said, "I'm referring to the green sweater you're wearing." Herm then answered, "Why shouldn't I wear it? My mother knit it for me." End of conversation.

On another occasion, Herm was MOD and seeing patients in the emergency room. It was a busy evening. A stack of a dozen or more patient records was on a table outside his examining room. After each patient was seen, Herm would pick the top record and call the next patient in. The records of newly arrived patients were placed on the bottom.

While examining one patient, Herm excused himself to respond to a knock on the door of his examining room. It was a brigadier general who asked imperiously, "When am I going to be seen, Captain Ortle?" Herm said, "I'm *Doctor* Ortle, and I'll see you as soon as your record comes to the top of the pile."

An hour or so later, the general was called in, fuming. He berated Herm for not bypassing the usual routine so that he, the general, could be seen sooner. The general kept referring to Herm as Captain Ortle. Herm kept correcting him—"I'm Doctor Ortle."

Finally, Herm had had enough. He said to the general, "I notice you have one star on your shoulder boards. That's a brigadier general, am I correct?" The general responded yes. Then Herm said, "A brigadier general—isn't that the lowest form of general?"

In spite of a number of such incidences, Herm received a commendation medal from the air force at discharge. The care of his patients had been exemplary. He returned to a professional life at an academic medical center in New Jersey and enjoyed a successful career.

Question:

1. *It is important that all patients be treated equally. How did you feel when you observed a physician speak to an uneducated patient in an arrogant or condescending manner or poor patients receiving lesser care than their middle- or upper-class counterparts?*

CHAPTER 47

Getting the Dose Right

Medicine is a science of uncertainty and an art of probability.

SIR WILLIAM OSLER

I was referred a young lawyer for evaluation of anemia. In the course of the visit, his fiancée asked to speak with me. She said she was concerned that her husband-to-be had never "made a pass" at her. She thought this unusual and wondered whether his anemia could be interfering with his sex drive.

Digging more deeply into the patient's history, it became clear that he had never had an erection. His muscle mass was less than his frame would have predicted. Further, he needed to shave only once every two to three days. Findings on physical examination included small testes and scrotum. A serum testosterone level was found to be very low, and gonadotropin-stimulating hormone (GSH) level was above normal. GSH is produced by the pituitary gland. It stimulates the production of testosterone. A low testosterone and high GSH level indicated that the end organs (testes) were unresponsive to pituitary stimulation. This is referred to as primary hypogonadism. Mild anemia, the reason for his referral to me, is a normal consequence of lack of testosterone.

When the patient and his fiancée returned for a visit after the tests were completed, I had an endocrinology colleague see him with me. It was explained to him that for normal sexual function, improved muscle mass and strength, and correction of anemia, it would be necessary for him to administer testosterone by injection every few weeks for the rest of his life. He readily agreed, and we began him on a cycle of testosterone every three weeks. The endocrinologist suggested that the frequency of spontaneous erections would be the best guide to the ultimate maintenance dose of the hormone.

Over the next three months, we increased the dose gradually. His anemia resolved, his muscle mass began to increase, and he began to shave every day. One day, when he returned for a routine visit, he had a black eye. We asked how this had occurred. He said that he was pulling into a parking space at the hospital parking lot and another man pulled in front of him and rammed his car into the open space. My patient was so angry that he got out of his car and accosted the other man. Punches were thrown and he received a black eye. My endocrinology colleague and I agreed that this incident indicated that he was on about the right dose of testosterone!

The patient subsequently married his fiancée and they moved to Washington, DC, to start a new life together.

Over the years, I often wondered how he was doing, what his subsequent life story was, whether he and his wife were happy together, if they had children, and how often he suffered a black eye.

Recall that learning is one of the key words in the definition of professionalism. Learning of the result of one's treatments is essential. Physicians need better follow-up systems to maintain contact with patients who have left their care. Only by following patients longitudinally can we understand the treatment's long-term effects.

If I were a surgeon, I would be interested in learning about the functional capacity and quality of life of the patients I operated on long into the future. For the patients that I provided with a new knee or hip, how many are now able to resume golf or tennis or skiing or walking without discomfort? How many did not fare as well and why not?

Question:

1. *Do you know of a health care system in this country that has the ability to track patients regardless of where the patient is, or when?*

CHAPTER 48

The President Is Dead

Assassination has never changed the history of the world.

BENJAMIN DISRAELI

I was the senior resident in charge of the emergency room at the Massachusetts General Hospital on November 22, 1963, the day that President John F. Kennedy was assassinated. That morning, I had returned home from the previous evening's 7:00 p.m. to 7:00 a.m. shift, which each of us six third-year residents carried for two months of the year.

My wife woke me at about 2:00 p.m. to break the news that the president had been shot and was dead. I was so groggy that I had difficulty comprehending what she was saying, but the enormity of the moment finally hit me. As I drove the twenty miles into the hospital that evening, I anticipated it would be a grueling night. By 7:00 p.m., as many as 70 percent of people in the United States were glued to their television sets. Some who were not were on their way to a hospital emergency room.

Shortly after I arrived for duty, a florid, forty-five-year-old Boston Irishman walked through the emergency room door, sweating and pale. I sat him down and asked about his symptoms. He could barely speak, mumbling a few words that I could hardly catch. I did hear him say he was panicked and felt faint. He had no chest pain or shortness of breath. He was not taking any medications and had no history of serious illness. I walked with him to an examining room and had him lie down. He was sweating profusely, his pulse was 140 and regular, and his blood pressure was 160/100. He indicated that his normal blood pressure was about 130/80.

I asked about when the feelings of panic and faintness began. He replied that it was after he'd been informed that the president had been assassinated. I gave him a strong sedative, and his symptoms and signs gradually abated. He was able to leave the emergency room and return home later that night.

During that evening of the tragic death of the president, I saw and sedated about twenty other Irish Catholic men, forty-five years of age, all with acute panic attacks. Their symptoms and signs were identical to those of the first patient I saw. They had identified with the president to such an extent that his assassination was as though someone had thrust a knife into their chests. Most required repeated sedation to relieve their symptoms.

This was a night I never would forget—relieving so many men of their angst over the president's death.

I have regretted not writing up this story and publishing it in the medical literature as a unique event, hopefully never to be repeated.

Question:

1. *Do you know of similar instances of acute panic attacks after the death of a famous person or an act of terrorism?*

PART FOUR

Key Challenges for Today's Medical Schools

The medicine of today is far different from that when most of the patient stories described in this book took place. The remarkable diagnostic technologies currently available such as CT, MRI, PET scanning, sophisticated diagnostic tests and non-invasive or minimally invasive procedures result in most diagnoses being made without having to be hospitalized. Most hospitalizations today are for complex treatments that cannot be performed in ambulatory settings. The pace of medicine is much faster, due, in part, to the almost exponential growth of medical knowledge and the vast array of treatments that can now cure or lead to improved function of patients with chronic disease. But new medical knowledge and technologies are developing faster than is our ability to utilize them wisely. Medicine and medical education thus face new challenges; balancing technology with humanism, educating for team care, utilizing new venues for learning and bringing quality of care to the highest possible level. The remainder of this book addresses some of these challenges, using a few stories to reinforce their importance.

CHAPTER 49

Technology and Humanism

The greatest mistake in the treatment of diseases is that there are physicians for the body and physicians for the soul, although the two cannot be separated.

PLATO

We need to be mindful that the marvels of medical technology don't displace the intensely personal aspects of health care. A few months ago, when visiting a very ill patient in the surgical ICU of one of the Boston hospitals, I was impressed with the electronic paraphernalia that the nurse was working with in the room of the patient. These included a computer screen where all the current lab data were displayed on a flow sheet, the overhead monitor with vital signs, EKG, pO2 readouts, and a poster-board-sized sheet of paper where the nurse was manually recording the data from both computers in serial fashion. Not very often did the nurse go to the bedside. For the moment, at least, he had become a prisoner of the technology, and the caring element was nowhere to be found.

Soon afterward, I visited one of the clinics of the hospital and observed a young primary care physician interacting with a patient in his office. I should say that he was interacting with the computer, not the patient. He too was off to the side, not looking at the patient, typing the responses to his questions into the electronic medical record. After the visit, he proudly stated that he never had to stay beyond normal clinic hours to complete notes on his patients. Well, technology had just secured another prisoner.

In a world where the need for humanism in patient care is ever more important, we, as role models, need to demonstrate to students, residents, and, if needed, other faculty how to avoid losing the art in the process of applying the science.

In 2003, a graduate of the medical school class of 1954, a respected internist in Rochester, was hospitalized at Strong Memorial Hospital. According to his wife, the resident assigned to his case was arrogant and rude and had informed the nurse that he was too busy to respond to her husband's complaint of pain. Later that day, the patient died, quite unexpectedly. Some years later, his wife attended what would have been his fiftieth medical school reunion and made the following comment:

"Medicine is intrinsically a very personal business. Healing is personal, and it often must extend beyond the wound to the psyche, and even to the patient's loved ones. The way medicine was practiced on Bernie has created far more wounds than it has healed. And as both the science and business of medicine march to ever greater heights, the 'art of medicine' withers and few will notice that in its path has been trampled a true and devoted healer."

These sad words remind us that even at a place steeped in patient-centeredness and caring, there are exceptions, and they need to be addressed whenever they are observed. Time for reflection will help. Dr. Michael Barry, a distinguished alumnus of the internal medicine residency program at Strong Memorial Hospital, told me recently that one of his "a-ha" moments during his residency was when he was caring for a terminally ill patient, writing orders for lab tests and x-ray procedures without much thought about the reason why, and not communicating with the patient or the family. He was totally preoccupied with tasks. Given the patient's condition, the tasks were irrelevant. He suddenly stopped and asked himself, "What am I doing, and why am I doing this?"

The insight he gained by asking these questions during the pressures of an exhausting residency program influenced his approach to the care of patients throughout the rest of his career. Indeed, he is known internationally for his work in promoting the role of the patient in medical decision-making.

How to make time for students and residents to reflect on their patient care experiences is a challenge that medical educators need to address. Role models can help by constantly demonstrating the attitudes and behaviors we expect of our residents.

Dr. Rita Charon, who directs the program in humanities and medicine and the clinical skills assessment program at the School of Medicine at Columbia University is doing just this. She has developed an innovative teaching method, a parallel chart system bringing literature and medicine together. She asks her students to keep a record of their own reactions to each case, their attempts to understand the patients' experiences, and the ways patients react to information given to them about their illnesses. It is a wonderful course, one that is highly valued by students. She now has established a PhD program in narrative medicine.

These strategies should apply equally to residents, some would say even more so. The fast pace of life during residency years tends to erode the very qualities we sought to instill in these physicians as students. Recently, Dr. James Cox, the head of radiation oncology at MD Anderson Cancer Center in Houston, told me that because his residents and fellows had lost the compassion and caring they had brought to medical school, he began to meet with them regularly to focus on the humanistic aspects of their professional lives. He has been delighted and reassured by their enthusiastic response. He needed only to give them permission to begin to discuss their feelings about their patients, their failures, their successes, and the uncertainties about long-term outcomes.

CHAPTER 50

Educating for Team Care

It takes a deep commitment to change and an even deeper commitment to grow

RALPH ELLISON

Patient care is increasingly dependent on good teamwork, from critical care at one end to the ambulatory management of patients with multiple chronic conditions on the other, the so-called patient-centered medical home. The team, not just the physician, takes responsibility for the patient. But effective teamwork doesn't just happen. First, it requires a change in the mindset of the physician from "I" to "we" and, second, an understanding and acknowledgment of each member's roles and abilities.

Here is the remark of a medical student after a few sessions of team-building with nursing and pharmacy students at the University of Minnesota: "When we discuss a case, I am thinking about the disease process and the medications. The pharmacy and nursing students might point out that those things may not matter because it's about systems, communication, and efficiency. When I stop talking and start listening to them, I learn from a very different perspective."

As the student implied, effective teamwork not only requires a change in mindset, it also requires good communication. Yet health professions students have little knowledge about or experience with communication, especially across professions. Here is a comment from an internationally recognized leader in critical care, Peter Pronovost from Johns Hopkins Hospital: *"When I was in medical school I spent hundreds of hours looking into a microscope yet I didn't have a single class that taught me communication and teamwork skills—something I need every day I walk into the hospital."xxv*

A few medical schools are now applying a new approach to their applicants to assess their communications skills, the multiple mini-interview, a series of brief interviews tied to case studies that require the student to think and communicate on his or her feet, each interview conducted by a different faculty member. This mini-interview initiative forces candidates to show they have the social skills to navigate a health care system in which good communication has become critical. The medical schools at Stanford, UCLA, and Oregon are among those using this approach.

The patient with a routine PSA test result of sixty-five who was not notified because there was no hand-off after a change of physicians and who showed up a year later with widespread bone metastases from his prostate cancer and the anesthesiologist who threw an epidural needle to the floor and stalked out of the room when the nurse confronted him about not using sterile technique, are real-world stories that might not have occurred if inter-professional learning for team care had been in effect when the physicians were in training.

We now live in a world where online learning, networking innovations, and simulation approaches are overcoming traditional barriers to inter-professional learning. So it is time to address the need for students from different health professions to learn about each other's skill levels and roles.

CHAPTER 51

New Venues for Learning

Sometimes we stare so long at a door that is closing that we see too late the one that is open.

ALEXANDER GRAHAM BELL

The Internet will make it possible for medical students to learn some elements of the curriculum more efficiently and free up time for the close personal interactions between student and teacher that we want so badly to preserve. One example is the Institute for Healthcare Improvement (IHI) in Cambridge, Massachusetts. It was the first to provide online learning opportunities for health professions students in content not usually addressed in the formal curricula of medical, nursing, and dental school, or not addressed in-depth. These include courses in communication, health policy, leadership, quality improvement, and safety. Facebook, YouTube, and other electronic venues are the vehicles for communication. The president of IHI at the time, Dr. Donald Berwick, and his team anticipated that a few hundred medical students would sign up for the newly opened school. The number was in the thousands, telling us something about subjects students are interested in that are not available at their medical schools.

MedU at the Institute for Innovative Technology in Medical Education at Dartmouth is another example on the same point. MedU is marketed "as the place where medical education knows no boundaries, empowering medical educators to collaborate directly to educate students whenever and wherever they are learning." This is indeed the case. Dr. Valerie Lang from the department of medicine at the University of Rochester School of Medicine was able to leverage her ideas about virtual patient cases for internal medicine clerkships through MedU so that online learning is now available for all students at every medical school in the country during their medicine clerkship. The acronym for her program is SIMPLE (Simulated Internal Medicine Patient Learning Experience).

Through these venues for more efficient learning, medical schools will be able to free up time for students to interact with master teachers, interactions that are essential if the learning objectives referred to in this book are to be met.

CHAPTER 52

Getting Serious About Quality

America's health care system is neither healthy, caring, nor a system.

WALTER CRONKITE

I spent some years working with Don Berwick and his staff at IHI. From my experience there, it's clear to me that academic medical centers (AMCs) still have a long way to go to achieve care of the highest order. AMCs believe they are leaders in quality and safety, but they need to address a number of goals that remain largely unmet: faculty who, by systematically measuring and improving their performance, serve as exemplars to students and residents; doing a better job of giving them the tools to measure and improve quality; public reporting of measures of quality; and the ability to track patients over time.

We can't expect students to be passionate about the level of their care, the monitoring of their performance, and their constant improvement if they don't see their teachers leading the way.

What happens to patients after they leave the hospital? Patients, particularly the elderly, are vulnerable during the immediate post-hospital period. Almost 20 percent of Medicare patients are re-hospitalized within thirty days after discharge. This problem is due largely to a lack of communication between the hospital-based physicians and the patient's primary care physician. Re-hospitalizations are reduced when systems are put into place to ensure a seamless transfer of responsibility for the patient's care. Post-discharge phone calls within forty-eight to seventy-two hours after transfer from hospital to home have been found to be effective in reducing the risk of readmission.

The lack of systems to track long-term outcomes is equally problematic. It has been about one hundred years since Dr. Amory Codman made the call for better information on patient outcomes.[xxvi] Codman was a surgeon at the Massachusetts General Hospital (MGH). He was the first American doctor to follow the progress of patients through their recoveries in a systematic manner. He kept track of his patients through "end result cards," which contained basic demographic data on every patient treated, along with the diagnosis, the treatment he rendered, and the outcome of each case. Each patient was followed up for at least a year to observe long-term outcomes. He also believed that all of this information should be made public so that patients could be guided in their choices of physicians and hospitals.

In 1914, the MGH refused his plan for evaluating surgical competence through this end-results program and the board of trustees took away his staff privileges there, only to reinstate them some years later when the board recognized the error of its ways.

Codman helped lead the founding of the American College of Surgeons and its Hospital Standardization Program, which later became the Joint Commission on Accreditation of Healthcare Organizations.

Here we are almost one hundred years later and most hospitals and health systems are still not able to track patients over time. Medical centers need to build patient tracking systems into their information infrastructure. Among other benefits, students and residents would learn the importance of long-term follow-up to monitor the effectiveness of care.

Author's Responses to Questions

Chapter 1: The Protective Parent

Questions 1 and 2: I told the mother that I was very uncomfortable with her request but that over the course of the weekend I would respect the request and present my concern to her physician when he returned. I took this approach because, having never seen the patient before, and thus never having established a doctor-patient relationship, I felt it would have been inappropriate for me to suddenly spring the diagnosis of acute leukemia on her. I supervised the patient's treatment until her physician returned, but I found it difficult to be a participant in this pattern of lying. I was disappointed that he had been willing to keep the patient in the dark about her disease. When he returned, he elected to continue the secrecy.

Question 3: The mother may have been fearful that her daughter would become seriously depressed to learn that she had leukemia. Further, for one reason or another, the mother may have harbored guilt over her daughter's illness.

Question 4: In most of the western world, people at age eighteen are considered adults and capable of making decisions on their own behalf.

Chapter 2: On Being Transparent

Question 1: Adverse events include medication errors, falls, wrong-side surgery, wound infection or infection at IV sites, mislabeled specimens, and wrong test or procedure. All are preventable.

Question 2: Any mistake that could result in harm should be shared with the patient or family.

Chapter 3: Not Enough Respirators

Question 1: There is no right answer here. The triage approach seems most appropriate to me, but age might be considered as well as family infrastructure. Neither race nor social status should be included in the decision-making.

Question 2: This is a difficult question. Unless a patient has indicated that no measures are to be undertaken to maintain life through artificial measures, such as a respirator, the physician is obligated to do everything possible on the patient's behalf. This would include the option of being transferred to a facility where there are sufficient resources to meet the needs of the patient if they are not available at the current site.

Question 3: Predictions may be accurate, but few physicians make decisions of this importance using statistics alone.

Chapter 4: Just One More Week

Question 1: This question does not have a yes or no answer. The wishes of the patient determine the approach to care. If he or she is not capable of decisions and has an advance directive, the directive takes precedence. In the absence of an advance directive, the spouse is next in line. If there is no spouse, the family must decide. Where there is no family, the medical team assumes the decision-making role. In this event, some physicians would respond yes to the question. Most would not and would focus on whatever treatment is necessary for the comfort of the patient.

Question 2: A frank discussion should occur between the patient and physician about the treatment options and the possible benefits and risks of each option. The patient's understanding of these options should be confirmed before obtaining written acceptance of the use of the experimental drug.

Chapter 5: Invasion of Privacy

Question 1: Virginity can be confirmed only if the hymen is intact. In many cases, however, the hymen will have ruptured by the age of fourteen as the result of trauma (i.e., bicycle riding) or the use of tampons.

Question 2: In response to the parents' request, I could have indicated that unless the patient's hymen is intact, it is not possible to determine whether she is a virgin. I could have indicated to the parents that they had invaded their child's right to privacy and asked them to leave. I could have acquiesced to their request on the grounds that their daughter was still a minor and therefore subject to their directives. I lied to the parents, principally because I was so angry that they had intercepted and read the letter to her. In retrospect, my behavior was not very professional. What if the patient had been in the early stages of pregnancy?

Chapter 6: Exposed

Questions 1 and 2: No response needed.

Question 3: Students often ignore evidence of poor care out of concern for their course grade. Incidents of poor care by a nurse or by a nonmedical staff member should be brought to the attention of the nurse manager. Where poor-quality care has been provided by a physician, the student may wish to discuss his or her concern with an advisor who is not directly involved in the care of the patient.

Chapter 7: Innovation

Question 1: First, determine whether the patient is conscious and breathing. If neither, check for the presence of a carotid pulse. If no pulse is found, straddle the patient, place the palm of one hand on the center of the chest and the other hand on top of the first. Push down firmly on the chest, compressing it about two inches. Perform about one hundred compressions a minute.

Most patients who have suffered a cardiac arrest are in ventricular fibrillation. A minority will have asystole. In either case, the purpose of cardiopulmonary resuscitation (CPR) is to partially restore blood flow to the brain and heart while awaiting the arrival of a defibrillator. Recently, studies of outcomes of patients after cardiac arrest show that it is not necessary to give artificial respiration while performing CPR. Indeed, the recovery is greater among those who were not given artificial resuscitation than in those who were.

Question 2: No response needed

Chapter 8: Confidentiality

Question 1: Fleck, trained in moral philosophy, suggests that the only circumstance where confidentiality may be excused is when there is an imminent threat of serious, irreversible harm, no alternative to avoiding the threat other than a breach of confidentiality, and proportionality between the threat of harm and the harm due to breaching confidentiality.[xxvii]

It wasn't until some years later that the AMA revised its code of ethics to permit breach of confidentiality if the patient is considered a threat to others or to himself.

Question 2: I believe so based upon the information provided above.

Question 3: Yes. One must remember, however, that the spouse of a substance abuser is a codependent and may be in denial.

Question 4: This is a good question, asked by a medical student. I did not inform the patient that I would be breaking confidentiality, but I should have.

Question 5: Not really. Assuring the airworthiness of the aircraft is as important as actions undertaken when the plane is aloft.

Chapter 9: Internship Hours

Question 1: The American College of Surgeons believes that the resident work-hour restriction results in less prepared physicians.

Question 2: Absent quantitative measures of performance, most physicians overestimate their decision-making ability after twenty-four to thirty hours of continuous work.

Chapter 10: Help Me Go

Questions 1–5: Good questions for group discussion.

Chapter 11: Mutiny

Question 1: If you feel that the patient is being harmed, you should bring your concern to the attention of the physician's supervisor.

Question 2: Unfortunately, this is a legitimate worry. I would go to a trusted mentor for advice.

Chapter 12: A Remarkable Response

Question 1: Over one hundred medicines currently in use are derived from plants. Plants are the original source material for as many as 40 percent of the pharmaceuticals in the US today. Examples include foxglove (digitalis), nightshade (atropine), colchicum (colchicine), rauwolfia (reserpine), mucuna (L-dopa), cinchona (quinine), and the yew tree (Taxol).

Chapter 13: Babies, Babies, Babies

Question 1: As a husband or father, I would be outraged.

Question 2: Attending physicians, additional residents, and nurses were available. We just never called them. As students and residents, we were considered weak if we called for help in handling our on-call responsibilities. Oversight and supervision were not what they are today. While I never experienced a serious incident for lack of help, some patients were undoubtedly discomforted by having to wait for our services.

You will undoubtedly encounter similar circumstances during your clinical years. How will you respond?

Chapter 14: The Giant Spleen

Question 1: Arguments in the patient record or in public must be avoided.

Question 2: A review of the published literature on the problem is in order to determine best practice. When no best practice has been established, a group of peers may be asked to render an opinion.

Question 3: The patient should be informed of the difference of opinion. Where best practice has not been determined, the patient should be encouraged to participate in the decision-making process.

Chapter 15: Legionnaires' Disease

Question 1: I should have been alert to this possibility.

Chapter 16: The General's Mother

Question 1: The patient indicated that her waist size had increased by two inches within a matter of weeks.

Question 2: Severe cardiac disease with right heart failure, portal hypertension from severe liver disease, and lymphatic obstruction from tumor or trauma are the most frequent causes of ascites.

Question 3: Liver or cardiac disease results in ascetic fluid that is the color of plasma (clear yellow). Involvement of the peritoneum from cancer usually results in somewhat cloudy yellow fluid. Milky white fluid is characteristic of lymphatic obstruction.

Chapter 17: Life-Changing Treatment

Question 1: This case taught us two important lessons. First, we should have anticipated a major change in the patient's physical and mental state and discussed it with both the patient and his wife. Second, given the number of years it must have taken to develop his level of hypothyroidism, we should have corrected the problem slowly, over a period of a year or more instead of in just three months.

Question 2: Other endocrine disorders such as hypopituitarism, chronic congestive heart failure, and cancer of the prostate (if treatment is needed at all).

Chapter 18: The Difficult Patient

Question 1: No response needed

Question 2: Show respect for the patient. Be nonjudgmental. Maintain a professional demeanor. If you need to let off steam, do so, but do it somewhere other than the patient's room.

Chapter 19: The Power over Life

Question 1. No response needed

Question 2: An injection of epinephrine gives immediate relief and is indicated in all patients with acute anaphylactic reactions and those with severe hives. Benadryl is commonly used to minimize itching. Corticosteroids provide longer-term relief from the allergic response.

Question 3: An allergy kit. It contains epinephrine for intramuscular injection (EpiPen, Twinject).

Chapter 20: Arrogance

Question 1: As per your experience.

Questions 2 and 3: Be honest in your response.

Chapter 21: Ad Hoc Survey

Question 1: You decide.

Chapter 22: Locked In

Question 1: No response needed

Question 2: Failure to listen to or elicit the patient's full story.

Chapter 23: The Abnormal EKG

Question 1: No treatment is indicated in patients with gallstones but without symptoms. In the ten years following the diagnosis of asymptomatic gallstones, only 25 percent will have required surgery.

Chapter 24: The Resident's Wife

Question 1: I would like to sit in on your response.

Chapter 25: Yes, Doctor

Question 1: Religious items such as a Bible or rosary beads; titles of books and magazines; articles of clothing and accessories; family pictures; writings on a wall calendar.

Chapter 26: Prelude to Suicide

Question 1: I should continue to talk. Remember that suicidal behavior is a cry for help. Patients with suicide intent may be deterred by helping them talk through their personal pain; witness people who have been "talked down" from a bridge or ledge of a building.

Chapter 27: Unexplained Findings

Question 1: The patient, while under observation, had been able to manipulate the rectal thermometer through rapid contraction and relaxation of anal muscles, resulting in a thermometer reading that reached 105 degrees! And she could accomplish this with so little body movement that the nurse, standing next to the bedside, would not notice it.

Question 2: That the physical examination and the results of all diagnostic tests and procedures were normal should raise a red flag.

Question 3: In humans, the nucleus of the red blood cell is extruded while it is still maturing in the bone marrow. The explanation for this is that until the nucleus is extruded, the red cell is not capable of deforming sufficiently to pass through tiny vascular spaces. Lower animals such as birds and chickens do have nucleated red cells circulating in the blood. In this case, when we presented our findings to the patient, she acknowledged that she had added some chicken blood to her urine sample.

Chapter 28: The Missing Teeth

Question 1: I confirmed with the patient that his findings were typical of past acute episodes. He defused the conflict between me and the other residents by refusing to consider surgery. As expected, after about forty-eight hours the symptoms went away almost as rapidly as they had appeared, and the patient was discharged home.

Here is a classic example of the need to listen to the patient and involve him or her in medical decisions. Patients with chronic or recurring illness almost always know the fine points of their disease better than do the physicians caring for them.

Questions 2& 3: For your response.

Chapter 29: The Certifying Exam

Question 1: For your response

Chapter 30: The Brioschi Man

Question 1: For your response.

Chapter 31: Overlooking the Obvious

Question 1: For your response.

Chapter 32: Life Anew

Question 1: For your response.

Chapter 33: Listen, Look, Feel

Question 1: An intra-abdominal tumor. Retroperitoneal masses such as a polycystic kidney or a retroperitoneal tumor are unlikely, as they would not have moved on inspiration.

Question 2: The presence of a splenic notch (hilum) on palpation.

Question 3: For your response .

Chapter 34: The Silent Tumor

Question 1: No response needed

Question 2: You would do well to discuss your concerns with a trusted advisor.

Chapter 35: The Murmur That Was

Question 1: Innocent murmurs are mid-systolic crescendo-decrescendo murmurs.

Question 2: Yes, unless there are other findings on auscultation of the heart.

Question 3: An echocardiogram.

Chapter 36: Nails

Question 1: Anemia, arthritis, scleroderma, superior mediastinal syndrome.

Chapter 37: Rusty Blood

Question 1: Hyper- and hypothyroidism, chronic organ failure (heart, liver, kidney), urinary obstruction (relieve by catheterization in hours, not minutes).

Chapter 38: Plugging Holes

Question 1: Cerebral hemorrhage, gastrointestinal bleeding.

Question 2: Aspirin inhibits platelet function. People with hemophilia are at much greater risk of bleeding if they take aspirin.

Chapter 39: Forty-Eight Pounds in Forty-Eight Hours

Question 1: The development of antibiotics such as penicillin resulted in a marked decrease in the complications of streptococcal infections from the 1940s onward.

Question 2: Simple bed rest and salt restriction would have resulted in a satisfactory initial diuresis. An orally administered diuretic would have resulted in greater control of further diuresis than the mercurial diuretic.

Chapter 40: A Life Taken

Question 1: No response needed

Chapter 41: Misinterpreting an Important Test

Question 1: There is no higher priority than to place an intravenous line to gain access to the circulation.

Chapter 42: About Courage

Question 1: No response needed

Chapter 43: Delicate Moments Faith

Question 1: No response needed

Chapter 44:

Question 1: There has never been a randomized control trial of the effectiveness of the Pap smear in reducing deaths from cervical cancer. A number of uncontrolled studies, however, have shown a substantial reduction in cancer deaths among those who have had regular Pap tests compared with those who did not.

The pelvic examination has not been shown to be helpful in screening for other disorders, such as cancer of the ovaries. The Pap smear should not be viewed in isolation from other screening tests in women. Tests for chlamydia and HIV infection are in order for many women, particularly adolescents.

Chapter 45: The Local Pharmacist

Question 1: No response needed

Chapter 46: The Brigadier General

Question 1: No response needed

Chapter 47: Getting the Dose Right

Question 1: The Veteran's Administration health system

Chapters 48-51: No questions

Epilogue

Patient stories will continue to serve as useful teaching material, but will the environment for medical education and clinical practice remain as exciting as the one I've described in this book? In recent years, physicians have pointed to loss of autonomy, burdensome paperwork, and patient demands for unneeded tests as principal reasons for dissatisfaction in medicine. Further, the speed with which new medical knowledge is generated and applied exceeds the ability of most physicians to keep up. Some physicians are advising young people not to go into medicine. Yet applications to medical school have not declined and the proportion of medical school graduates who elect training in primary care is increasing.

Trends in how medicine is organized, delivered, and paid for will reduce dissatisfaction with medical practice, though it may take a generation to achieve. Increasingly, physicians are joining hospitals and health systems as salaried employees, giving up independence in order to escape the burden of managing an office practice. Hospitals are now restructuring to become health systems, adding skilled nursing facilities, visiting nurse services, hospice care, pharmacy services, retirement communities, and the like. These health systems are preparing to become accountable care organizations, accepting the responsibility for providing high-quality health care services to a population of patients. Physicians and administrators in the health system are working to coordinate services in ways that better meet the needs of patients, the so-called patient-centered medical home.

Payment for medical services will change as well. The current fee-for-service system is fragmented, promotes overutilization of services, and generates unnecessary costs, including high administrative costs, for both providers and health insurance companies. A single bundled payment for an episode of illness or for a given patient for a year of care will relieve health systems and insurance companies of an enormous administrative burden and reduce the tendency to over-utilize services. Further, a single global payment will provide an incentive for physicians and other providers to use efficient ways to meet patient needs. The expanded use of the phone and e-mail, for example, are efficient ways of communicating that are greatly underutilized under the fee-for-service payment system.

Finally, as pointed out in chapter 49, the move to team-based care will give physicians the opportunity to spend more time with their complex patients. Nurse practitioners and non-physician providers will be able to expand their services to the extent of their skills.

These changes will make it possible to achieve the goals of twenty-first-century health care, so well-articulated in the 2001 report of the Institute of Medicine as care that is safe, effective, timely, efficient, equitable, and patient-centered.[xxviii] Will this goal be achieved?

About the Author

Throughout his fifty-nine year career in medicine, Paul Griner has been a teacher and mentor to countless medical students, residents, and fellows, faculty, and practicing physicians. He is a professor of medicine emeritus at the University of Rochester School of Medicine and Dentistry and was a consultant at the Massachusetts General Hospital, senior lecturer at Harvard Medical School, and consultant to the Institute for Healthcare Improvement (IHI) in Cambridge, Massachusetts. He is the author or coauthor of one hundred thirty journal articles, book chapters, and books on subjects in clinical medicine, medical education, and health policy. He is a member of the Institute of Medicine of the National Academy of Sciences and was president of a number of national medical organizations, including the American College of Physicians. He continues to be a mentor to many.

Notes

(Endnotes)

i. Francis W. Peabody, "The Care of the Patient," *JAMA* 88 (1927): 877–882.

ii. Ibid.

iii. Benedict Martina, MD, et al., "First Clinical Judgment by Primary Care Physicians Distinguishes Well Between Non-Organic and Organic Causes of Abdominal or Chest Pain," *Journal of General Internal Medicine* 12 (1997): 459–465.

iv. P. L. Stillman et al., "An Assessment of the Clinical Skills of Fourth Year Medical Students at Four New England Medical Schools," *Academic Medicine* 65 (1990): 320–326.

v. Richard A. Deyo, "Cascade Effects of Medical Technology," *Annual Review of Public Health* 23 (2002): 23–44.

vi. Louis Brandeis, *Business: A Profession* (Boston: Small Maynard, 1914).

vii. R. M. Epstein and E. M. Hundert, "Defining and Assessing Professional Competence," *JAMA* 287 (2002): 226–235.

viii. University of Washington School of Medicine, *Bioethics in Medicine* (Seattle: University of Washington School of Medicine, 1998).

ix. A. Cote, "Telling the Truth? Disclosure, Therapeutic Privilege, and Intersexuality in Children," *Health Law Journal* 8 (2000): 199–216.

x. Steve S. Kraman and Ginny Hamm, "Risk Management: Extreme Honesty May Be the Best Policy," *Annals of Internal Medicine* 131 (1999): 963–967.

xi. Elihu Schimmel, "The Hazards of Hospitalization," *Annals of Internal Medicine* 60 (1964): 100–110.

xii. Institute of Medicine, *Crossing the Quality Chasm: A New Health System for the 21st Century* (Washington, DC: National Academies Press, 2001).

xiii. D. T. Baran, Paul F. Griner, and M. R. Klemperer, "Recovery from Aplastic Anemia After Treatment with Cyclophosphamide," *New England Journal of Medicine* 295 (1976): 1522–1523.

xiv. Eisenstadt v. Baird, 405 U.S.438 (1972).

xv. Robert Sharpe, "The Impact of Prolonged Continuous Wakefulness on Resident Clinical Performance in the Intensive Care Unit," *Critical Care Medicine* 38 (2010): 766–770.

xvi. A. L. Back, J. I. Wallace, et al., "Physician-Assisted Suicide and Euthanasia in Washington State: Patient Requests and Physician Responses," *JAMA* 275 (1996): 919–925; D. A. Asch, "The Role of Critical Care Nurses in Euthanasia and Assisted Suicide," *New England Journal of Medicine* 334 (1996): 1374–1379.

xvii. Asch, "Role of Critical Care Nurses," 1374–1379.

xviii. Michael J. Barry, "Shared Decision Making: Informing and Involving Patients to Do the Right Thing in Health Care," *Journal of Ambulatory Care Management* 35 (2012): 90–98.

xix. Jerome Groopman, *How Doctors Think* (New York: Houghton Mifflin, 2007).

xx. Robert Petersdorf and Paul Beeson, "Fever of Unknown Origin: Report of 100 Cases," *Annals of Internal Medicine* 70 (1969): 864–868.

xxi. William L. Morgan and George L. Engel, *The Clinical Approach to the Patient* (Philadelphia: W. B. Saunders, 1969).

xxii. W. Bean, "Some Notes of an Aging Nail Watcher," *International Journal of Dermatology* 15 (1976): 225–230.

xxiii. Bernie S. Siegel, Love, *Medicine and Miracles: Lessons Learned About Healing from a Surgeon's Experience with Exceptional Patients* (New York: Harper and Row, 1986).

xxiv. Robert Ader and Nicholas Cohen, "Behaviorally Conditioned Immunosupression," *Psychosomatic Medicine* 37 (1975): 333–340.

xxv. Peter Pronovost and Eric Vohr, Safe Patients, Smart Hospitals (New York: Hudson Street Press, 2010).

xxvi. E. A. Codman, "The Product of a Hospital," *Surgery, Gynecology & Obstetrics* 18 (1914): 491–496.

xxvii. Leonard Fleck and Marcia Angell, "Please Don't Tell," *Hastings Center Report* (1991): 39.
xxviii. Institute of Medicine, *Crossing the Quality Chasm*.

AAA 1800 222 4357

Made in the USA
Lexington, KY
11 December 2012